COMMUNITY:
A HUMAN BECOMING PERSPECTIVE

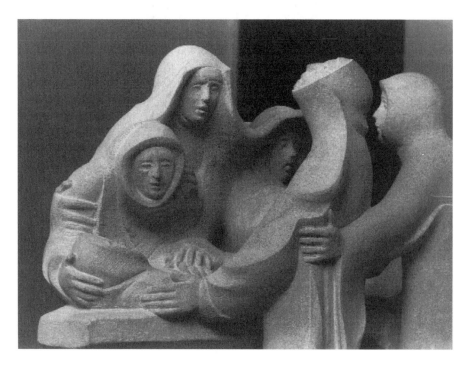

Reprinted with permission of Sisters of the Order of Saint Benedict, Saint Benedict's Monastery, St. Joseph, MN.

Community
Sculpture by Joseph O'Connell
1927–1995

COMMUNITY:
A HUMAN BECOMING PERSPECTIVE

Rosemarie Rizzo Parse, RN, PhD, FAAN
Professor and Niehoff Chair
Loyola University Chicago

JONES AND BARTLETT PUBLISHERS
Sudbury, Massachusetts
BOSTON   TORONTO   LONDON   SINGAPORE

World Headquarters
Jones and Bartlett Publishers
40 Tall Pine Drive
Sudbury, MA 01776
978-443-5000
info@jbpub.com
www.jbpub.com

Jones and Bartlett Publishers Canada
2406 Nikanna Road
Mississauga, ON L5C 2W6
CANADA

Jones and Bartlett Publishers International
Barb House, Barb Mews
London W6 7PA
UK

Library of Congress Cataloging-in-Publication Data

Parse, Rosemarie Rizzo,
    Community : a human becoming perspective / Rosemarie Rizzo Parse.
      p. cm.
    Includes bibliographical references and index.
    ISBN: 0-7637-1564-6
    1. Nursing—Philosophy. 2. Quality of life. I. Title.
    [DNLM: 1. Philosophy, Nursing. 2. Health. 3. Quality of Life. WY 86 P266c 2003]
    RT84.5 P355 2003
    610.73'01—dc21

                                                                    2002043092

Acquisitions Editor: Penny M. Glynn
Production Manager: Amy Rose
Associate Production Editor: Karen C. Ferreira
Associate Editor: Karen Zuck
Production Assistant: Jenny L. McIsaac
Senior Marketing Manager: Alisha Weisman
Associate Marketing Manager: Joy Stark-Vancs
Manufacturing Buyer: Amy Bacus
Cover Design: Alj Mary, The Iron Rose Complex, Inc.
Interior Design: Carlisle Communications, Ltd.
Composition: Chiron, Inc.
Printing and Binding: Malloy Incorporated
Cover Printing: Malloy Incorporated

Printed in the United States of America
07 06 05 04 03   10 9 8 7 6 5 4 3 2 1

CONTENTS

9   Stories of Courage and Confidence: An Interpretation
With the Human Becoming Community Change Concepts   131

Debra A. Bournes

10   Community: Glimpses of the Possibles   147

Rosemarie Rizzo Parse

CONTRIBUTORS

Debra A. Bournes, RN, PhD
Director of Nursing—New Knowledge and Innovation
University Health Network, Toronto, Canada

Sandra Schmidt Bunkers, RN, PhD, FAAN
Associate Professor of Nursing
Augustana College, Sioux Falls, South Dakota

William K. Cody, RN, PhD
Professor and Chair
Family & Community Nursing Department
University of North Carolina at Charlotte, North Carolina

Human community is a living dialogue of many worlds of meaning.

—From Adrian van Kaam, Bert van Croonenburg, and Susan Muto, The Emergent Self, 1968, p. 70, Wilkes-Barre, PA: Dimension Books, Inc.

That which is, already has been; that which is to be, already has been.

Ecclesiastes 3:15 RSV

PREFACE

There is a notable shift in the focus of human science disciplines with regard to the idea of community. Scholars in the human sciences are turning attention to community as more than a location or group with similar interests. The purpose of this book is twofold: (a) to set forth definitions and examples of original community change concepts and processes arising from the human becoming school of thought; and (b) to expand the meaning of community beyond location and interest-related groups.

In this book there are chapters offering glimpses of traditional community definitions found in the general and nursing literature. There is a chapter on community in the arts with a human becoming perspective. Community, from a human becoming perspective, is a oneness of human-universe connectedness incarnating beliefs and values. The major human becoming community change concepts (moving-initiating, anchoring-shifting, pondering-shaping) are elaborated upon through processes that incarnate everyday situations related to health and quality of life. Examples of the community change processes are included along with three chapters by Parse scholars who live the art and sciencing of human becoming with community. Also explicated in this work are Parse research method findings interpreted in light of the human becoming community change concepts.

Faculty, graduate and undergraduate students, researchers, and practitioners of nursing and other human science disciplines will find this work an alternative to the traditional way of viewing community. This will be especially helpful in gaining an in-depth understanding of human experiences of health and quality of life. With the evolution of the human-universe process as basic to the human sciences, this book is set forth to promote dialogue among human science scholars as they become more concerned with community as a unitary phenomenon.

CHAPTER 1

COMMUNITY: GLIMPSES OVER TIME

ROSEMARIE RIZZO PARSE

In this first decade of the twenty-first century, the idea of community is emerging as a central concern in a variety of scholarly discourses. This is particularly true in the health-related disciplines, such as nursing, which are struggling to emerge from the domination of medicine. What is of concern here is that there is no one definition of community, and the traditional definitions do not capture the essences of the emerging human sciences, now becoming important as guides in healthcare delivery. Newer definitions are on the horizon; for example, Parse (1999), Nancy (as cited in Pontbriand, 2000), and Wheatley and Kellner-Rogers (1998) posit definitions of community that are consistent with each other and with the emerging human sciences. Parse says that community is a oneness of human-universe connectedness incarnating beliefs and values. Nancy (as cited in Pontbriand, 2000) says that he does not use the term community since he believes it is an exclusive term; he sees community as a "universal being-with" (p. 16). Wheatley and Kellner-Rogers (1998) say that communities are "webs of relationships" (p. 10). While these definitions are central to the explication of human becoming community concepts, the focus of this book, it is important to recall some of the traditional definitions of community. To that end, a glimpse of meanings of community over time are presented here.

Diverse meanings that have evolved over time in local, global, and virtual arenas are from the foci of the various social disciplines concerned with the nature of community. Since the foci reflect the beliefs and values of the scholars of a discipline, there is no one definition of the term community that is compatible with the different paradigmatic views. Here, the author presents some of the most widely known definitions from a variety of general sources.

Perhaps the most recognized early work on community is that of Ferdinand Tönnies (1888/1988), who developed the concepts of *Gemeinschaft* (community) and *Gesellschaft* (society) consistent with his interest in how people relate to each other, and how relationships are vehicles for social change. The definition of *Gemeinschaft* is fellowship, a mutuality best expressed in families and neighborhoods with common bonds and multiple obligations. This definition represents a local view of community and is still widely used.

Robert Ezra Park (1936/1988), in an ecological study of urban life in Chicago, defined community more broadly as a plant, animal, or human involved in "a process of competitive cooperation" (p. 27). This competitive cooperation is a "system of relations between the species ... involved in an orderly process of change and development" (p. 30) through competition, dominance, and succession. Park says that the ecological concepts of competition, dominance, and succession differ in human communities from those of plants and animals, since the human environment is not biologically fixed, nor is the social organization of humans developed by instinct. A community of humans is composed of two levels: "a symbiotic society based on competition and a cultural society based on communication and consensus" (p. 33). According to Park, human communities from an ecological perspective include "(1) population, (2) artifacts (technological culture), (3) customs and beliefs (nonmaterial culture), and (4) the natural resources—that maintain at once the biotic balance and the social equilibrium" (p. 34). Competition and consensus are cyclical processes that move people in ways that create social change. Park's definition is viable today in the social sciences.

In 1955, Hillery reported on a literature review conducted to discover the extent of consensus on the definitions of community. He analyzed 94 anthropological and sociological definitions and discovered only one consistent theme throughout, that "people are involved in community" (p. 119). Other characteristics that he found to be common in the published definitions are self-sufficiency; a common life; the possession of common ends, means, and norms; a consciousness of homogeneity; a collection of institutions; and localism (Hillery, 1955).

Norton Long (1958/1988), a political scientist, utilized a game analogy when speaking of a local community or territorial system. For Long, "the local community ... is an order in which expectations are met and functions performed" (p. 41) through structured group activities. These group activities "that coexist in a particular territorial system can be looked at as games." The human "is both a game-playing and game-creating animal ... and through games and activities ... he [she] achieves a satisfactory sense of significance and a meaningful role" (p. 42). Long speaks of "a political game, a banking game, a contracting game, a newspaper game, a civic organization game, an ecclesiastical game, and many others" (p. 42). However, Long believes it is the social game that provides linkages among the others and encourages cooperation toward shared hopes and dreams in community.

Stonewall (1983) found it problematic to define community at all, since too many "different social phenomenons [sic] have been called communities ... cities, institutions, neighborhoods, villages, hotels, prisons, minority groups, religious organizations, military establishments, trade unions and professions" (p. 2), depending on the researcher's perspective. Stonewall set out to find a definition that would have "both inclusive and exclusive qualities that ... [would] distinguish ... [the] concept from others" (p. 2). Not only was there disagreement about what should be included in the definition, there was little consensus as to which elements were most important. Keeping this in mind, Stonewall defined community as "people interacting in a specific time and place" (p. 1). From the three essential elements of people, time, and place, Stonewall identified five theories of community to help make sense of the diverse definitions: human ecology, structural functionalism, conflict, sociopsychological approaches, and network-exchange analysis (p. 1).

Most recently, Mason (2000), a political scientist, proposed two concepts of community: an ordinary concept and a moralized concept. Unique to Mason's definition of both concepts is the fact that he not only defines community from both perspectives but also conceptually defines key phrases in each. For Mason, the ordinary community is "constituted by a group of people who share a range of values, a way of life, identify with the group and its practices, and recognize each other as members of the group" (p. 20). Mason said that ordinary community consists of a collection of people who pursue similar goals. Further, he said that

a way of life is a set of rule-governed practices, which are at least loosely woven together and which constitute at least some central areas of social, political and economic activity ... involv[ing] cooperative activities.... To identify with a group and its practices ... is to commit oneself to it in a way that normally involves endorsing its practices and seeking to promote its interests, whilst regarding one's own well-being as intimately linked to its flourishing. (p. 23)

Mason's moralized definition of community incorporates all of the ordinary concepts of community plus three further conditions: "solidarity between its members ... mutual concern ... [and] no systematic exploitation or systematic injustice" (p. 27). According to Mason, it is possible that an ordinary community may not be a moralized community. The ordinary definition of community serves as a means of identifying people's allegiances and behaviors. The moralized definition serves to "condemn social and political arrangements or praise them" (p. 34).

Postmodern perspectives of community are found with the works of Wilkinson (1972), Cohen (1985), Hinchman and Hinchman (1997), Carey and Frohnen (1998), and Wheatley and Kellner-Rogers (1998). Kenneth Wilkinson (1972), a sociologist, defines community as "a social field" (p. 51). With Wilkinson's definition of *field*, a unitary perspective of community begins to surface in the literature.

> Fields are emergent in the sense that they differ from the sum of the characteristics of their components. They are dynamic in that they are constantly changing. "Unbounded" means literally without boundaries—fields shade into one another and must be distinguished according to their core properties rather than according to the characteristics of their perimeters. A field is holistic in the sense of having a configurational or systemic unity. (Wilkinson, 1972, p. 51)

Wilkinson (1972) says a social field is "a process of interaction through time, with direction toward some more or less distinctive outcomes and with constantly changing elements and structure" (p. 51). As the social field is emergent, dynamic, and unbounded, outcomes cannot be predicted as multiple possibilities arise at any one moment.

Cohen (1985) defined community somewhat differently as "members of a group of people having something in common with each other, which distinguishes them in a significant way from the members of other putative groups" (p. 12). This definition suggests a simultaneous inclusion as well as exclusion of people in the formulation of a community. The inclusion in a community depends on "commonality of forms (ways of behaving) whose content (meanings) may vary considerably among its members" (p. 20). Cohen suggests that community is a matter of meaning arising from the community members' perspectives, which cannot be defined or assessed objectively.

For Hinchman and Hinchman (1997), community is also concerned with meanings. It is "constituted by narratives.... They explain a group to itself, legitimate its deeds and aspirations, and probe important benchmarks for nonmembers trying to understand the group's cultural identity" (p. 235). The narratives comprise meaning moments chosen by community members as they communicate their perceptions of themselves to others within and without the community. Community comes about with communication, which is the process of sharing experiences with day-to-day discourse and artistic and scientific expressions.

For Carey and Frohnen (1998), sharing experiences is fundamental to community. They believe commonality of experiences is the singular most significant aspect of community, since they define community as "one in which the members share something in common, something important enough to give rise to fellowship or friendship and sustain it" (pp. 1–2). For them, a community will not only not exist but also cannot be vital and functional unless the community evolves around "experiences, practices, and beliefs that are important enough to bind the members to one another ... such that they are sharers of a common fate" (p. 2).

Wheatley and Kellner-Rogers (1998) elaborate further on community, and speak of communities arising from a paradox, two dimensions of human existence, individualism and connectedness. They report that satisfaction with one dimension is generally at the expense of the other, since the very act of belonging to a community involves a choice of forfeiting at least some autonomy. The authors do allow for another perspective. In choosing how one lives, "freedom gives rise to the boundless diversity of the planet ... an individual exercises its freedom continuously ... free to decide what to notice, what to invest with meaning" (p. 11). "We create ourselves by what we choose to notice" (Wheatley, 1999, p. 12). As an individual chooses the *other,* connectedness arises, and "over time, individuals become so intermeshed in this process of coevolving that it becomes impossible to distinguish the boundary between self and other" (Wheatley & Kellner-Rogers, 1998, p. 12). This is "when a community knows its heart, its purpose for being together" (p. 16). Thus, for Wheatley and Kellner-Rogers, communities are "webs of relationships ... [where] diverse individuals live together in ways that support both the individual and the entire system ... [as] new capabilities and talents emerge from the process of being together ... coevolving" (pp. 10–11).

Hesselbein, Goldsmith, Beckhard, and Schubert (1998) speak of global communities of the future as "interdependent and diverse, embracing differences, releasing energy, and building cohesion.... Those living within each community define all community" (p. xi). Zobel de Ayala (1998) says that "inclusion and participation" (p. 263) "[will drive] human beings [to continue] to form communities that excite their sense of obligation and commitment.... They will prefer to belong rather than to secede" (p. 271).

Traditional modern perspectives of community, then, arise with the definitions of Tönnies (1888/1988), Park (1936/1988), Hillery (1955), Long (1958/1988), Stonewall (1983), and Mason (2000). Community from this perspective is considered objective, measurable, and concerned with relationships, change, symbiosis, localism, cooperation, and the commonality of interests and goals. Postmodern perspectives of community arise with definitions by Wilkinson (1972), Cohen (1985), Hinchman and Hinchman (1997), Carey and Frohnen (1998), and Wheatley and Kellner-Rogers (1998), who address social fields, dynamism, unity, communication, individual perspectives, meaning, interdependence, universality, freedom, and paradox. In the next chapter, some of these ideas and the human becoming perspective are discussed in relation to community and the arts.

References

Carey, G., & Frohnen, B. (Eds.). (1998). *Community and tradition: Conservative perspectives on the American experience.* Lanham, MD: Rowman & Littlefield.

Cohen, A. (1985). *The symbolic construction of community.* Chichester, England: Ellis Horwood.

Hesselbein, F., Goldsmith, M., Beckhard, R., & Schubert, R. (Eds.). (1998). *The community of the future*. San Francisco: Jossey-Bass.

Hillery, G. (1955). Definitions of community: Areas of agreement. *Rural Sociology, 20,* 112–123.

Hinchman, L., & Hinchman, S. (1997). *Memory, identity, community: The idea of narrative in the human sciences*. Albany: State University of New York Press.

Long, N. E. (1988). The local community as an ecology of games. In R. Warren & L. Lyon (Eds.), *New perspectives on the American community* (pp. 41–51). Chicago: The Dorsey Press. (Reprinted from *American Journal of Sociology*, Vol. 64, pp. 251–261, 1958)

Mason, A. (2000). *Community, solidarity, and belonging: Levels of community and their normative significance*. Cambridge, England: Cambridge University Press.

Park, R. E. (1988). Human ecology. In R. Warren & L. Lyon (Eds.), *New perspectives on the American community* (pp. 26–34). Chicago: The Dorsey Press. (Reprinted from *American Journal of Sociology*, Vol. 42, pp. 1–15, by R. E. Park, 1936)

Parse, R. R. (1999). Community: An alternative view. *Nursing Science Quarterly, 12,* 119–124.

Pontbriand, C. (2000). Jean-Luc Nancy/Chantal Pontbriand: An exchange. *Parachute, 100,* 14–31.

Stonewall, L. (1983). *Country life, city life: Five theories of community*. New York: Praeger.

Tönnies, F. (1988). Gemeinschaft and gesellschaft (C. Loomis, Trans.). In R. Warren & L. Lyon (Eds.), *New perspectives on the American community* (pp. 7–15). Chicago: The Dorsey Press. (Original work published 1888)

Wheatley, M. (1999). Consumed by fire or fire: Journeying with T. S. Eliot. *Noetic Sciences Review, 48* (April–July), 11–15.

Wheatley, M., & Kellner-Rogers, M. (1998). The paradox and promise of community. In F. Hesselbein, M. Goldsmith, R. Beckhard, & R. Schubert (Eds.), *The community of the future* (pp. 7–18). San Francisco: Jossey-Bass.

Wilkinson, K. (1972). A field theory perspective for community development research. *Rural Sociology, 37*(1), 43–52.

Zobel de Ayala, J. A. (1998). Anticipating the community of the future. In F. Hesselbein, M. Goldsmith, R. Beckhard, & R. Schubert (Eds.), *The community of the future* (pp. 261–271). San Francisco: Jossey-Bass.

CHAPTER 2

COMMUNITY: GLIMPSES FROM THE ARTS

ROSEMARIE RIZZO PARSE

The idea of community is alive in the arts. Honour and Fleming (1982), in their comprehensive work, *The Visual Arts: A History*, indicate that the content, style, and subject matter of Western art from ancient Greek and Roman times portrayed community through a concentration on religious icons and the aristocracy. It was not until the Renaissance and after that the arts were connected with common people, their interrelationships, their possessions, and events of the day. Throughout history the arts have engaged individuals and groups, cocreating lifestyles and illustrations of community as a oneness of interconnections, affirming beliefs and values. According to Chantal Pontbriand (2000a), editor of *Parachute* (a journal of contemporary art), the idea of community is and always has been important in the art scene. Among other things, artworks show a search for identity in relationships with others, and a concern for balance between individual and group portrayals, all of which reflect various community profiles as a oneness of interconnections. Pontbriand says community is not a totality but exists as the intersubjective space between and among persons. Dissanayake (2000) concurs when she says that the arts are a manifestation of human connectedness with others and the universe, and, further, she claims that they are intrinsic to human existence. Dissanayake (2000) says, "To take the arts seriously is to rediscover routes to belonging, meaning, and competence" (p. xv). Consistent with this idea is Miller's (2001) view that art is now shifting even more toward integration with community. He uses the example of the artist Linda K. Johnson, who in creative configurations plants vegetables on a median strip in downtown Portland, drawing community into art.

The importance of community and the arts also arises as a concern among philosophers. Pontbriand (2000b) interviewed French philosopher Jean-Luc Nancy regarding community and the arts. According to Pontbriand (2000a), "Art is ... a method of thinking" (p. 9). Nancy (as cited in Pontbriand, 2000b) stresses that the nonexclusive community is open and infinite. He says, "I don't like to use the term community" (p. 15). He prefers to speak of "being-in-common or being-with" (p. 15), avoiding the exclusive connotation of the word community. Nancy says, "'I' am, from the very onset, 'with' (near) those who precede my birth and those who follow my death" (p. 15). Here Nancy shares a view of art as a human interlinking, which is similar to Parse's (1981, 1998) notion of the all-at-once presence of predecessors, contemporaries, and successors as community. This idea is embodied in *Six Degrees of Separation*, the play by John Guare (1990) and the movie, directed by Fred Schepisi (Schepisi & Milchan, 1998), in which the playwright shows how one person is connected to and through others to all other persons.

The presentation of the arts in this chapter is not intended to be exhaustive but, rather, only a glimpse of meanings of community with selected artists and forms of art viewed with the human becoming lens. For this glimpse there is a brief discussion of a critic's view, three artists, a photographer, a number of paintings, one play, and three films.

Artists as Community: Critics and Painters

Artists live community as they reflect and cocreate society. For example, Craven (1996) says that Robert Motherwell's writings reveal his beliefs that progressive artists as community are on the margin of society, yet their art is inextricably connected with societal changes. Craven reports that although Motherwell's concerns were mainly with ethics and values in art, he saw a profound connection among artists as a group and their influence on the shifting value priorities in society. This notion is consistent with Daniels' (2001) view. An example of artists as community can be seen in Daniels' work when he writes of Vincent van Gogh's deep concern with community, contradicting the idea of van Gogh as an isolated loner. Van Gogh had a vision of art as a source of hope for society, and of a "brotherhood of painters joined in the pursuit of shared beliefs" (Druick & Zegers, 2001, p. 1). Van Gogh invited Paul Gauguin to join him in Arles, France, to initiate such a brotherhood. The two worked together at the Studio of the South in Arles for only 9 weeks but cocreated new and different ways of painting. When Gauguin left for the tropics to build his own brotherhood of artists, both he and van Gogh extended their own works separately, but they were forever connected in light of the moments they shared. Their ideas and lived community rippled as both artists worked with other artists seeking new themes and techniques. From their community cocreations came pointillists such as Georges Seurat, Camille Pissarro, and others. These artists shared ideas and values as community, affirming their beliefs in the art movement of the times and by making contributions to societal change in light of their art.

Twentieth-century pop artist Andy Warhol cocreated a different community, focusing on cultural images bringing to the fore the ideas, people, and commodities of the moment (Ratcliff, 1983), such as repetitive pictures of Elizabeth Taylor, Jacqueline Kennedy, Marilyn Monroe, and Campbell's® soup cans. Warhol's work was pivotal in moving art to another level in that it was uniquely connected with everyday reality. The images he portrayed brought forth the idea of community, not only in the unique arrangement of the work, but even more so in what it symbolized to the observer in terms of the images and meanings in media shared almost automatically. Danto (1999) said that the pop art dramatized by Warhol's work created the interesting problem of distinguishing philosophically "between reality and art when they resembled one another perceptually" (p. 5). Danto believes that Warhol achieved an unprecedented unity in that his art and life were one. "He turned the world we share into art, and turned himself into part of that world, and because we are the images we hold in common with everyone else, he became part of us" (Danto, 1999, p. 83). Warhol's contributions, and those of his disciples, cocreated new societal traditions and new conceptualizations of the nature of art and art's relation to people.

These observations of three artists' lives offer just a glimpse of how the artist cocreates community as an indivisible, ever-changing human connectedness. The individual is community; the group is community; the universe is community.

Artists as Community: The Photographer

St. Gelais (2001) analyzes the photographic work of Dutch artist Rineke Dijkstra in light of the current genre of documentary portraiture. St. Gelais says that Dijkstra's work depicts a "community of solitudes" (p. 18). He photographs typical individuals with universally recognizable features—alike in some ways, yet different in others. This idea connects in some way Parse's (1981, 1998) paradox of conformity–non-conformity in originality, the being alike and different all-at-once. St. Gelais says that in Dijkstra's photographs there is a "coming into being" (p. 21) of community at a moment suggesting only a glimpse of what was before and after the freeze frame. Photographers like Dijkstra cast their artists' eyes upon a scene and take snapshots, capturing a moment of community as a oneness of interconnections.

Art as Community: The Paintings

Paintings by all artists in some ways depict cocreated values of community that arise from the artist's own belief system. Artists pour into their paintings visions of community, telling stories of their times. For example, Rembrandt's famous work *The Night Watch* (1642) depicts a Dutch militia entering the street. It is a community in alert expectation cocreating the value priorities of the moment. This community is in stark contrast to Renoir's (1881) in *The Luncheon of the Boating Party*, which portrays a segment of a French community (Figure 2.1). The focal point shows people engaging in leisurely relaxation and joyful conversation, a community living the cocreated values arising with the situation. Picasso's well-known *Guernica* (1937) shows a different community, one of inhumanity and horror, explicating his view of the global political environment during the Spanish Civil War. *Guernica* is a deeply moving piece depicting cocreated pain with the connecting and separating with the war. Van Gogh (1885) depicts another dark time in his solemn painting *The Potato Eaters*, which shows a community of families and neighbors held together during a famine.

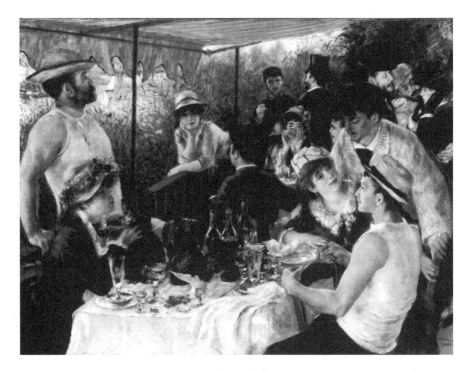

Figure 2.1 Renoir, Pierre Auguste, **Luncheon of the Boating Party**, 1880–81, oil on canvas, $51\frac{1}{4} \times 69\frac{1}{8}$ inches. Acquired 1923, The Phillips Collection, Washington, DC. Reprinted with permission.

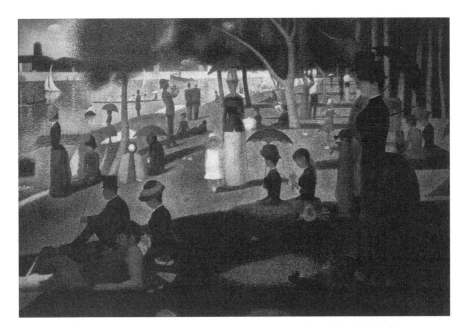

Figure 2.2 Seurat, Georges, French, 1859–1891, **A Sunday on La Grande Jatte—1884**,
1884–86, oil on canvas, 207.6 × 308 cm, Helen Birch Bartlett Memorial Collection,
1926.224, reproduction ©2002 The Art Institute of Chicago. Reprinted with permission.

In a more joyful painting, A *Sunday on La Grande Jatte* (1884–1886), pointillist
Georges Seurat, an art-scientist, depicts people and animals enjoying a relaxing afternoon by the water in a moment of communion-aloneness (Herbert,
1991) (Figure 2.2). Camille Pissarro's *The Market at Gisors* (1899) portrays an
everyday scene in the marketplace, as community is shown with women rest-
ing and talking. His *Avenue de l'Opera: Morning Sunshine* (1898) shows a community of eager people bustling in an effort to get somewhere. The somewhere
can only be imagined by the observer, who enters the painting with a personal
history cocreating yet another community.

These and many other widely recognized paintings call attention to the
embeddedness of community as an interconnection of human values in the
arts. There are realms upon realms of meanings of community in the paintings.
The artist's tacit-explicit history, as depicted in the painting, is there with the
meaning of the painting to the observer, who arrives at the painting with a personal history as well. The engagement with art is community with community
with community with community.

Art as Community: Plays and Films

"The play's the thing/Wherein I'll catch the conscience of the King" (Shake-speare, act II, scene ii, lines 633–634). Shakespeare's words echo down the years portending the idea that the play catches attention and engages people, depicting meanings for the moment. The play as community shines forth as a communing with at many realms, that is, the writer with the director and actors, and the actors with the observers. All are engaged, not only with each other, but also with the histories that each brings to the moment of con-tact and beyond. Multiple communities surface multiple meanings. The glimpse here of community in a play is with Samuel Beckett's (1954) *Waiting for Godot*. The play depicts community lived through two players engaging in shared moments in the wait for a god who never arrives. The characters move with and away from each other through dialogue that discloses and hides glimpses of their histories, the disappointments of the now, and hopes for what is yet-to-be. Beckett's views shape community as lived with individual and others.

Like the play, film is a moving medium, carrying the viewers along in a story of community. Two films that uniquely depict community as multidimensional are *Being John Malkovich*, directed by Spike Jonze (Jonze & Kaufman, 1999), and *A Beautiful Mind*, directed by Ron Howard (Grazer & Howard, 2001). In *Being John Malkovich*, various persons enter the brain portal of John Malkovich and play out a meaning moment, blurring the boundaries of human connectedness (Pettman, 2001). The people entering John Malkovich cocreate unpredictable opportunities constitutive of their values and beliefs of the moment. The com-munity is constantly shifting as characters enter and exit, cocreating their histories anew while living their many realms of knowing.

Another example of community as living many realms of knowing was made explicit in *A Beautiful Mind* (Grazer & Howard, 2001). The film portrays the life of Nobel Prize winner John Forbes Nash Jr., whose reality was coconstituted with others whose identities were not made visibly available to his family or contemporaries. Community was clearly portrayed as a oneness of human connectedness. Yet another community was depicted in *The Shawshank Redemption* (King, 1982; Marvin & Darabont, 1994). In this film, directed by Frank Darabont, imprisoned men cocreated patterns of relating, incarnating their histories in living with the rules, being forced to be like others and yet struggling to be unique. This is similar to Parse's (1981, 1998) notion of the par-adox conforming–not conforming. During moments in the movie of explicit nonconformity, the central theme of hope surfaces again and again, as the men take risks in rare moments of rebellion. An interesting note on living commu-nity, as depicted in this film, was clearly illustrated when men who had been incarcerated for more that half their lives were released; these men continued living the prison community, incarnating who they were becoming. Their living of the prison community while moving with a free society was slowly integrated with different experiences as they cocreated community anew.

Community is the individual and, thus, with groups of individuals; it is clearly not a location. It is cocreated with the universe as lived over time—all that is, has been, and will be. It is a oneness of interconnectedness lived uniquely, incarnating values and beliefs of personal histories in the fleeting moments of ever-changing becoming.

The glimpses of community and the arts (the critics, the artists, the photographer, the artworks, the play, and the films) reflect a concern for individuality, universality, meaning, and paradox. They are perspectives on community somewhat alike and, yet, different from those articulated in the previous chapter on general literature and in the next chapter, where glimpses of community from the nursing literature are presented.

References

Beckett, S. (1954). *Waiting for Godot*. New York: Grove Press.

Craven, D. (1996). Aesthetics as the ethics in the writings of Robert Motherwell and Meyer Schapiro. *Archives of American Art Journal, 36* (1), 25–32.

Daniels, J. (2001). Vincent van Gogh and the painters of the petit boulevard: St. Louis Art Museum. *Art News, 100* (2), 197.

Danto, A. (1999). *Philosophizing art: Selected essays*. Berkeley: University of California Press.

Dissanayake, E. (2000). *Art and intimacy: How the arts began*. Seattle: University of Washington Press.

Druick, D. W., & Zegers, P. K. (2001). *Van Gogh and Gauguin: The studio of the south*. New York: Thames and Hudson.

Grazer, B. (Producer), & Howard, R. (Director). (2001). *A beautiful mind* [Motion picture]. United States: Universal Studios and DreamWorks Pictures.

Guare, J. (1990). *Six degrees of separation*. New York: Random House.

Herbert, R. L. (1991). *Seurat*. New York: Metropolitan Museum of Fine Art.

Honour, H., & Fleming, J. (1982). *The visual arts: A history*. New York: Harry N. Abrams, Inc.

Jonze, S. (Director), & Kaufman, C. (Writer/Co-Executive Producer). (1999). *Being John Malkovich* [Motion picture]. United States: USA Films.

King, S. (1982). *Rita Hayworth and the Shawshank redemption in different seasons*. New York: Penguin.

Marvin, N. (Producer), & Darabont, F. (Director/Writer). (1994). *The Shawshank redemption* [Motion picture]. United States: Columbia Pictures and Castle Rock Entertainment.

Miller, A. (2001). The growing impact of environmental art. *Artweek, 32* (4), 17–18.

Parse, R. R. (1981). *Man-living-health: A theory of nursing*. New York: Wiley.

Parse, R. R. (1998). *The human becoming school of thought*: A perspective for nurses and other health professionals. Thousand Oaks, CA: Sage.

Pettman, D. (2001). "In the fine underwear of our minds": Love and community in the age of globalism. *Parachute, 101*, 64–71.

Picasso, P. (1937). *Guernica* [Oil on canvas, 349.3 × 776.6 cm]. Madrid: Prado Museum.

Pissarro, C. (1898). *Avenue de l'opera: Morning sunshine* [Oil on canvas, 65 X 81 cm]. Philadelphia: Private Collection.

Pissarro, C. (1899). *The market at Gisors* [Painting, 52 × 63 cm]. Retrieved May 5, 2002, from http://www.vincent.nl/gallery/paintings/0700/a722.htm.

Pontbriand, C. (2000a). [Introduction to the issue]. *Parachute, 100*, 6–11.

Pontbriand, C. (2000b). Jean-Luc Nancy/Chantal Pontbriand: An exchange. *Parachute, 100*, 14–31.

Ratcliff, C. (1983). *Warhol*. New York: Abbeville Press.

Rembrandt. (1642). *The night watch* [Painting]. Amsterdam: Rijksmuseum.

Renoir, P.-A. (1881). *The luncheon of the boating party* [Oil on canvas, 129.5 × 172.7 cm]. Washington, DC: The Phillips Collection.

St. Gelais, T. (2001). Rineke Dijkstra: A community of solitudes. *Parachute, 102* (April–June), 14–31.

Schepisi, F. (Producer/Director), & Milchan, A. (Producer). (1998). *Six degrees of separation* [Videorecording]. Santa Monica, CA: MGM/UA Home Video.

Seurat, G. (1884–1886). *A Sunday on la grande jatte* [Oil on canvas, 208 × 308 cm]. Chicago: The Art Institute of Chicago.

Shakespeare, W. (1978). Hamlet. *The annotated Shakespeare: The tragedies and romances*. Vol. 3. Edited by A. L. Rowse. New York: Clarkson N. Potter, Inc./Publishers.

van Gogh, V. (1885). *The potato eaters* [Oil on canvas, 82 × 114 cm]. Amsterdam: Vincent van Gogh Museum.

CHAPTER 3

COMMUNITY: GLIMPSES FROM THE NURSING LITERATURE

ROSEMARIE RIZZO PARSE

Community has always been of interest to nursing, but mostly as a location, and has been described conceptually in the traditional paradigm of the discipline. The traditional paradigm of nursing is the totality paradigm, where the human is viewed as a biopsychosocialspiritual being, either adapting to, or manipulating the environment. Health is viewed on a continuum. Healthcare providers and societal norms determine whether a person is healthy or unhealthy, goals are delineated in terms of maintenance of the health state or restoration to a normal health state, and practice outcomes are measured quantitatively (Parse, 1987, 2000). Since the totality paradigm is the predominant paradigm, most definitions of community in the nursing literature reflect this view.

The American Nurses Association (1986) adapted the World Health Organization's definition of community in its *Standards of Community Health Nursing Practice*. Community is "a social group determined by geographical boundaries and/or common values and interests.... It functions within a particular social structure, exhibits and creates norms and values, and establishes social institutions" (p. 17). Community defined in this way is traditionally the basis for community health nursing and public health nursing practice. In 1999, The Quad Council of Public Health Nursing Organizations developed the *Scope and Standards of Public Health Nursing Practice*, distinguishing the difference between community nursing and public health nursing. Even though the focus of these two entities is somewhat different, both are circumscribed by population and geographic location.

Consistent with this view, system theory, which became popular in nursing in the early 1980s, is still very attractive for use in community health nursing. It focuses on the interactions of the parts of a system, provides "a useful framework for viewing individuals, families, and communities and for viewing interrelationships among these systems as they influence health" (Helvie, 1981, p. 5). A system can be open or closed. It is hierarchical, has boundaries that exchange energy with other systems, and has a feedback loop mechanism. Since all of these characteristics of a system suggest that no single factor is responsible for the state of a system, it appears that multicausal factors underlie a particular state. In community health nursing, the systems most commonly referred to are the body system and the organizational system, both of which require balance (health). The role of the community nurse from this perspective is to assist the system(s) either to maintain balance or regain balance through primary prevention, or secondary and tertiary interventions.

Spradley and Allender (1996), in their text on community health nursing, refer to the traditional notion of community as a geographic relational group of people with common interests forming "the basis for a sense of unity or belonging" (p. 5). The authors refer to a "community of solution ... [whereby] a group of people ... come together to solve a problem that affects all of them" (p. 6). This community of solution may not be a new idea, as it appears to have as its base, social change theory, similar to Tönnies' (1888/1988) view of community: families and neighborhoods with bonds and obligations as boundaries.

Shields and Lindsey (1998), unlike Spradley and Allender (1996), suggest moving away from the traditional nursing view of the *community as context*, which focuses "on the environment in which a person lives" (p. 24), to the view of "community as resource ... dynamic and changing ... [addressing] capacities and strengths ... [and] community as client [that] encourages nurses to view community as a whole, to identify health issues that transcend the community, and to perceive the community as a unit of practice" (p. 25). As such, community health promotion requires nurses "to move beyond these traditional conceptualizations to explore the meaning of community as a relational experience of being in community.... [It is] more than simple involvement in relationships with other people.... It denotes an ontology, a way of being that permeates throughout people's lives" (p. 26). The authors state their belief that health promotion, as a relational experience of being in community, should advance four "new patterns of practice: (1) listening and critical reflection; (2) participatory dialogue and critical questioning; (3) pattern emergence and recognition; and (4) movement to action.... The components are often interwoven, iterative, synergistic, and fluid" (pp. 29–30).

Smith-Campbell (1999) similarly defined community as "a plurality of persons when a common geopolitical locale, tie, or affinity is shared" (p. 406). The term "plurality suggests that persons exist as part of the whole, are joined together to exist and function together to contribute to the emergence of the whole" (p. 406). Smith-Campbell says this definition is rooted in Giorgi's concept of primacy of relationships within the human experience, and that "human beings are a part of the world, communities are ... connected with the environment" (p. 406).

The above definitions from the nursing literature are mostly consistent with the totality paradigm in nursing and are basically similar to traditional definitions in the general literature specified in chapter 1. In contrast to these views stand the definitions with postmodern perspectives from the general literature by Wilkinson (1972), who says community is a holistic field; Hinchman and Hinchman (1997), who say community is a phenomenon concerned with meanings shared through discourse and artistic and scientific expressions; Wheatley and Kellner-Rogers (1998), who say community is a *web of relationships*; and Nancy (as cited in Pontbriand, 2000), who says that community is a *universal–being with*; and, from the nursing literature, by Shields and Lindsey (1998), who say community is a relational experience. These few definitions are ontologically more consistent with the simultaneity paradigm in nursing and, thus, with Parse's (1999) definition, from the human becoming school of thought, of community as a oneness of human-universe interconnectedness.

The human becoming school of thought specifies that humans are multidimensional in mutual process with the universe, living all-at-once the was, the is, and the not-yet (Parse, 1981, 1998, 2001). Health is the process of becoming (Parse, 1990, 1998), and quality of life is defined as the meaning a person or group gives to life at the moment in cocreation with the universe (Parse, 1994). The art and sciencing of human becoming focuses on lived experiences. Based on this ontology, then, the definition of community is an alternative to the traditional definitions with several distinctions in meaning.

Community from Parse's (1999) view is a oneness of human-universe interconnectedness incarnating unique beliefs and values. This perspective is grounded in the philosophical assumptions and principles of human becoming (Parse, 1981, 1992, 1995, 1997, 1998, 2001) (see Tables 3.1 and 3.2).

From a human becoming perspective, the human and universe are in mutual process cocreating what is, thus cocreating community. *Cocreation* refers to the coconstitutive nature of the human-universe mutual process; this means that all that is arises with the constituents of a situation. Who an individual human being is is always in cocreation with all that is the universe. Humans are unitary. They are indivisible, unpredictable, and ever-changing beings who choose value priorities imaged in mutual process with the multidimensional universe. *Multidimensionality* refers to the boundaryless infinity of explicit-tacit knowings lived all-at-once. The explicit-tacit knowings are interwoven interconnections surfacing meanings of the moment. The meanings given to situations cocreate personal histories that incarnate health. Individuals bring to each event their personal histories. These are the realities that are the individuals' languaged imaged values, cocreated with predecessors, contemporaries, and successors. A community (individual or group),

Table 3.1. ASSUMPTIONS OF HUMAN BECOMING

Assumptions About the Human and Becoming	Assumptions About Human Becoming
The human is coexisting while coconstituting rhythmical patterns with the universe.	Human becoming is freely choosing personal meaning in situation in the intersubjective process of living value priorities.
The human is open, freely choosing meaning in situation, bearing responsibility for decisions.	Human becoming is cocreating rhythmical patterns of relating in mutual process with the universe.
The human is unitary, continuously coconstituting patterns of relating.	Human becoming is cotranscending multidimensionally with emerging possibles.
The human is transcending multidimensionally with the possibles.	
Becoming is unitary human-living-health.	
Becoming is a rhythmically coconstituting human-universe process.	
Becoming is the human's patterns of relating value priorities.	
Becoming is an intersubjective process of transcending with the possibles.	
Becoming is unitary human's emerging.	

Note: From *The Human Becoming School of Thought* (pp. 28–29), by R. R. Parse, 1998, Thousand Oaks, CA: Sage Publications, Inc. Copyright 1998 by Sage Publications, Inc. Adapted with permission.

Table 3.2. PRINCIPLES OF HUMAN BECOMING

Principles	Concepts of the Principles
Structuring meaning multidimensionally is cocreating reality through the languaging of valuing and imaging.	*Imaging* is reflective-prereflective coming to know the explicit-tacit all-at-once.
	Valuing is confirming–not confirming cherished beliefs in light of a personal worldview.
	Languaging is signifying valued images through speaking–being silent and moving–being still.
Cocreating rhythmical patterns of relating is living the paradoxical unity of revealing-concealing and enabling-limiting while connecting-separating.	*Revealing-concealing* is disclosing–not disclosing all-at-once.
	Enabling-limiting is living the opportunities-restrictions present in all choosings all-at-once.
	Connecting-separating is being with and apart from others, ideas, objects, and situations all-at-once.
Cotranscending with the possibles is powering unique ways of originating in the process of transforming.	*Powering* is the pushing-resisting process of affirming–not affirming being in light of nonbeing.
	Originating is inventing new ways of conforming–not conforming in the certainty-uncertainty of living.
	Transforming is shifting the view of the familiar-unfamiliar, the changing of change in coconstituting anew in a deliberate way.

Note: From *The Human Becoming School of Thought* (pp. 35–58), by R. R. Parse, 1998, Thousand Oaks, CA: Sage Publications, Inc. Copyright 1998 by Sage Publications, Inc. Adapted with permission.

then, is coconstituted with all the personal histories of those present. What arises as the distinctiveness of community incarnates the diverse meanings that individuals with their histories give to the moment. Although the evolution of community over time has recognizable patterns of constancy, diverse patterns surface as personal histories change with new experiences. Whether the community is an individual, a city, a group, or a galaxy, there is continuous change, cocreating patterns of constancy-diversity. Thus, community is an ever-changing process, not a static geographical location. (Parse, 1999, pp. 119–121. Copyright 1999 by Sage Publications, Inc. Adapted by permission of Sage Publications, Inc.)

Human-universe patterns are rhythmical, paradoxical, unrepeatable flowing processes. Community patterns of relating are chosen ways of revealing-concealing, as all decisions enable and limit all-at-once the connecting-separating of people, ideas, objects, and events. Rhythmical patterns cocreate community interconnectedness. Transcending, moving beyond the moment with possibles, is powering human-with-universe, while originating different ways of becoming in multidimensional, moment-to-moment, day-to-day, and year-to-year transforming. Community (individual or group) pushes and resists while conforming and not conforming in living the certainty and uncertainty of the familiar-unfamiliar. Community emerges with the hopes and dreams of constituents as they struggle and leap beyond, expanding horizons. Community is the structured meanings arising with imaged values lived out in languaging, as paradoxical rhythms of revealing-concealing and enabling-limiting emerge with connecting-separating. Community transforming unfolds with powering the originating of new ways of becoming. (Parse, 1999, pp. 119–121. Copyright 1999 by Sage Publications, Inc. Adapted by permission of Sage Publications, Inc.)

Community, however broad, wide, and deep, is incarnated with the unique patterns of constancy-diversity by which it is recognized. From the human becoming perspective, then, the galaxy, for example, is community, in that there are patterns in the arrangements of planets and stars with their inhabitants that reflect a constancy and diversity that can be recognized. The constituents of the galaxy form rhythmical patterns that cocreate the galaxy itself. The world, countries, states, cities, groups, families, and individuals are at one with the galaxy community, yet each of these entities has unique rhythmical patterns that make each a community, and all of these entities coconstitute each other. These are multidimensional webs of interconnectedness. It may not be difficult to recognize most of these entities as community, since they are clearly cocreated with more than one. But how is an individual community? An individual is community in that s/he selectively engages in face-to-face meetings; dialogues with printed materials; communicates through the galaxy-wide web; and imagines with people, ideas, objects, and events, abiding with predecessors, contemporaries, and successors multidimensionally all-at-once. Even before an individual's conception, the parents live imaginings that are incarnated with that individual's becoming. So, no engagement with another is without community. The individual is community, the family is community, the group is community, the world is community, the galaxy is community. (Parse, 1999, pp. 119–121. Copyright 1999 by Sage Publications, Inc. Adapted by permission of Sage Publications, Inc.)

This human becoming perspective of community, an ever-changing incarnated interconnectedness cocreated with all that is, is in stark contrast with most traditional definitions presented in earlier chapters in this book. The major difference is in the ontological base of the human becoming school of thought. In the next chapter, the author sets forth the conceptualizations born out of this ontology, offering a different way of understanding and living community.

References

American Nurses Association. (1986). *Standards of community health nursing practice.* Kansas City, MO: Author.

Helvie, C. O. (1981). *Community health nursing: Theory and process.* Philadelphia: Harper & Row.

Hinchman, L., & Hinchman, S. (1997). *Memory, identity, community: The idea of narrative in the human sciences.* Albany: State University of New York Press.

Parse, R. R. (1981). *Man-living-health: A theory of nursing.* New York: Wiley.

Parse, R. R. (1987). *Nursing science: Major paradigms, theories, and critiques.* Philadelphia: Saunders.

Parse, R. R. (1990). Health: A personal commitment. *Nursing Science Quarterly, 3,* 136–140.

Parse, R. R. (1992). Human becoming: Parse's theory of nursing. *Nursing Science Quarterly, 5,* 35–42.

Parse, R. R. (1994). Quality of life: Sciencing and living the art of human becoming. *Nursing Science Quarterly, 7,* 16–21.

Parse, R. R. (Ed.). (1995). *Illuminations: The human becoming theory in practice and research.* New York: National League for Nursing Press.

Parse, R. R. (1997). The human becoming theory: The was, is, and will be. *Nursing Science Quarterly, 10,* 32–38.

Parse, R. R. (1998). *The human becoming school of thought: A perspective for nurses and other health professionals.* Thousand Oaks, CA: Sage.

Parse, R. R. (1999). Community: An alternative view. *Nursing Science Quarterly, 12*, 119–121.

Parse, R. R. (2000). Paradigms: A reprise. *Nursing Science Quarterly, 13*, 275–276.

Parse, R. R. (2001). *Qualitative inquiry: The path of sciencing.* Sudbury, MA: Jones and Bartlett.

Pontbriand, C. (2000). Jean-Luc Nancy/Chantal Pontbriand: An exchange. *Parachute, 100*, 14–31.

Quad Council of Public Health Nursing Organizations. (1999). *Scope and standards of public health nursing practice.* Washington, DC: American Nurses Association.

Shields, L. E., & Lindsey, A. E. (1998). Community health promotion nursing practice. *Advances in Nursing Science, 20* (4), 23–36.

Smith-Campbell, B. (1999). A case study on expanding the concept of caring from individuals to communities. *Public Health Nursing, 16,* 405–411.

Spradley, B. W., & Allender, J. (1996). *Community health nursing: Concepts and practice* (4th ed.). Philadelphia: Lippincott.

Tönnies, F. (1988). Gemeinschaft and gesellschaft (C. Loomis, Trans.). In R. Warren & L. Lyon (Eds.), *New perspectives on the American community* (pp. 7–15). Chicago: The Dorsey Press. (Original work published 1888)

Wheatley, M., & Kellner-Rogers, M. (1998). The paradox and promise of community. In F. Hesselbein, M. Goldsmith, R. Beckhard, & R. Schubert (Eds.), *The community of the future* (pp. 7–18). San Francisco: Jossey-Bass.

Wilkinson, K. (1972). A field theory perspective for community development research. *Rural Sociology, 37* (1), 43–52.

CHAPTER 4

HUMAN BECOMING COMMUNITY CHANGE CONCEPTS

ROSEMARIE RIZZO PARSE

Community, from a human becoming perspective, is a unitary phenomenon, indivisible, unpredictable, and ever-changing (Parse, 2002). It is an incarnation of unique patterns of the coevolving life histories of diverse entities. Histories are cocreated multidimensionally with predecessors, contemporaries, successors, ideas, objects, and events.

In this chapter, the author sets forth a new set of community concepts arising from the human becoming school of thought (Parse, 1981, 1998). Community concepts from this view are unitary paradoxical rhythms of change: moving-initiating, anchoring-shifting, and pondering-shaping. These rhythms arise in all day-to-day relationships as new meanings unfold with shifting patterns in cocreating what is possible.

The discussion that follows grounds the human becoming change concepts and processes with the three principles of human becoming and is followed by illustrations of situations of living community. All of these situations are stories incarnating the meaning of health and quality of life as lived with community from a human becoming perspective.

Moving-Initiating Community Change

Moving-initiating is a cocreated paradoxical rhythm of community change. It is discarding and creating all-at-once, incarnating the value priorities of community, whether community is an individual or group. In this case the discarding and creating is related to barriers and constraints that are not moved without initiating new ones. Community barriers are reality structures, the cocreated meanings of the moment that are discarded and created to conform or not conform with traditional value priorities. Meanings change with different community experiences; thus, there is both certainty and uncertainty arising with changing the familiar-unfamiliar. How a change is viewed is consistent with the meanings given to the unfolding moments. The moving-initiating of barriers discloses and hides the value priorities of community, and the chosen opportunities and restrictions language imaged possibles, as meaning surfaces in different ways of connecting-separating. There is a unique pushing-resisting process arising with community that incarnates the risk of affirming a new way of being with the uncertainty that lies with the tacit of the not-yet-explicitly-known.

Moving-initiating community change has nine processes. They were conceptualized during the author's experience at the Checkpoint Charley Museum in Berlin, Germany, near the Brandenburg Gate. Checkpoint Charley was the main ingress to and egress from East and West Berlin from 1961 to 1989. The museum contains pictures and artifacts depicting the ways people attempted to cross the border by land, water, and air. The author synthesized

---

Table 4.1. DEFINITION AND PROCESSES OF MOVING-INITIATING COMMUNITY
CHANGE

Moving-initiating is a cocreated paradoxical rhythm of community change.

Tunneling is digging under, piercing the depths in cocreating situations for deliberately earthing and unearthing ideas, objects, and events.

Driving is forging directly with intensity in cocreating shifting patterns of diversity.

Laddering is climbing multidirectionally in planning and executing strategies.

Boating is steering while navigating the calm-turbulence of shifting waves and winds, harnessing moments of buoyancy, yet always with ambiguity.

Swimming is gliding with diverse currents in keeping afloat with sureness-unsureness.

Submarining is immersing in a high pressure enveloping at great depth with the shifting of what is known and not yet known explicitly.

Ballooning is drifting vigilantly with the pattern of the whole in a buoyant surgence-release, while shifting winds cocreate the unexpected.

Motorflying is propelling persistently with the gravity of weaving winds.

Swinging is soaring in undulating suspension with gusts of shifting winds in swingshifting to and fro in a bold leaping beyond.

---

the ideas when dwelling with the meaning of the situation and named the conceptualizations as described here. The definitions of these processes illuminate the moving-initiating change concept of the human becoming view of community (see Table 4.1).

Tunneling

Tunneling is digging under, piercing the depths in cocreating situations for deliberately earthing and unearthing ideas, objects, and events in moving-initiating community change. Community tunnels in a variety of ways by exposing and covering up happenings; thus, in all that arises with community, there is the disclosed and hidden. In moving-initiating change both should be considered. The value priorities of community are languaged in what is earthed and unearthed, incarnating the meaning of the situation. All earthing and unearthing enables and limits ways of connecting-separating. Tunneling is a subtle pushing-resisting arising in affirming community situations in the face of potential disregard. The covering and disclosing of the familiar-unfamiliar is a way of cocreating conformity–non-conformity with the certainty and uncertainty in living community.

Illustration of Tunneling

Alice appeared before a board of nursing to request that her inactive license be reinstated to active status. Alice had placed her license on inactive status after she was fired from her job for allegedly stealing drugs from her workplace. After her arrest, Alice entered into a plea agreement with the court system, served minimal jail time and an extended probation, and then made the decision to seek reinstatement of her nursing license. This was the second time she had been involved with the court system for alleged theft of drugs. Upon submitting her application for reinstatement of her license, she was required to answer a series of questions regarding whether or not she had ever been convicted, pled guilty, or received a suspended imposition of sentence for anything other than a minor traffic violation. Alice answered yes, and the state board began investigating. A date was scheduled for Alice to appear before the board.

Alice's appearance was that of a very professional, articulate young woman who related her perspective of the situation. She explained that she was the victim of a conspiracy at her employment setting, where she refused to participate in a surgical procedure that she believed was an abortion. When it was brought to the attention of the administration that there were drugs missing from the workplace, she was reported to the police. Although she maintained that she did not steal the drugs, she chose to enter into a plea bargain whereby she pled guilty to a felony and received a lesser sentence than she would have otherwise. She said she did this because she was afraid that she would have ended up in jail for an extended period of time if the case had gone to trial. Additionally, there was evidence presented to the board by a woman claiming that controlled substances were missing from her home after Alice visited.

The board members, after hearing all of the facts, including the meaning of the situation for Alice, decided that the theft issue had been handled by the court system, but the board members believed they could not ignore the concern that there was a chemical dependency issue. They voted not to reinstate her license until she had completed 1 year in an assistance program for health professionals.

From the time Alice had entered into the plea bargain and placed her license on inactive status, she was living the tunneling process as her way of cocreating meaning. She was all-at-once earthing-unearthing details about her own situation. By entering into the plea agreement, Alice was simultaneously earthing-unearthing the details that she wanted disclosed and those she wanted hidden. By putting the license on inactive status, earthing it, Alice was trying to protect it, yet her action was what cocreated the unearthing of the details of the case. Her decision to try to reactivate her license resulted in her admission of a conviction in the past, and the state board began an investigation to dig further into the facts—to pierce the depths of what happened. As the details began to be unearthed, Alice attempted to cover them as much as possible by weaving the conspiracy story. Some of the board members thought her conspiracy story was plausible. Alice's explanation both earthed and unearthed details, adding clarity in some ways, yet confusing or obscuring the actions of the court in other ways.

The tunneling arose as a digging and piercing process; the more Alice told, the more the board dug to understand what was happening. Meanings changed moment to moment as the revealing-concealing shifted. The board heard Alice's perspective in the situation that was cocreated by Alice, the board, the court, the other person who shared information, the workplace, and all of the predecessors, contemporaries, and successors and ideas therewith. The decision made by the board was cocreated by Alice's telling a story that they did not believe. The value priorities of this community were cocreated with new meanings surfacing in all that happened in moving-initiating community change.

Another Illustration of Tunneling

When Bill arrived to assume his new position as director of the intensive care unit, he found a place much different from what he had expected. Bill had been told that an accreditation visit was anticipated in 6 months but that preparation was well underway and there was not much to complete. However, as he came to know the community of healthcare providers, he learned that the policy and procedure book had not been updated for several years, there were no organized education records for staff members, and there was a pet mouse in the report room of the intensive care unit.

Bill found himself digging under to discover the real story. Staff members carried out their nursing care in ways unfamiliar to him. If a shift was about to end, leaving on time was valued higher than assuring that patients in the department were being cared for safely. Standards were vague, and healthcare was substandard from Bill's perspective. As Bill pierced the depths of the department's struggles, he learned that staff members did not have a clear understanding of the mission and philosophy of the hospital or their own values. Bill invited discussions about personal values and values that were important to the intensive care unit community. The group discussed ways to be with physicians who demanded the firing of staff nurses who made decisions that in the physicians' opinions were not supportive of medicine. There was enormous energy being expended when discussing matters with irate physicians who were personally affrontive and verbally destructive.

As issues were unearthed, ideas were earthed. Staff members began to support one another. They cocreated, without staged plans, to be with one another when physicians were disruptive to the flow of patient care. For example, when Dr. Jones would lose his temper and shout in loud and disturbing ways, the nurses circled around him in silence until his demeanor changed.

Meanings changed as value priorities changed. The unearthing and earthing continued as the entire demeanor of the department was transformed. Staff members began to realize that education and record keeping were important. Preparing for accreditation was a priority, and change was necessary. The accreditation report was positive, but Bill knew the group had a long way to go; looking good on paper was one thing, but being an effective, tight-run ship that provided quality patient care was quite another. Tunneling was ongoing during Bill's tenure in the position, as he had to be deliberate in all his actions, and communicate with many to hear their struggles and cocreate meanings anew in moving-initiating community change.

Driving

Driving is forging directly with intensity in cocreating shifting patterns of diversity in moving-initiating community change. Forging directly is cocreating meaning with pushing-resisting in a quickening pace in affirming being amid the potential of disregard. The intensity of cocreating anew arises with conforming and all-at-once not conforming with traditional ways as the certainty and uncertainty of change unfolds. There are a variety of ways of forging directly in shifting patterns of change that are revealed-concealed in the way community is speaking–being silent and moving–being still. Driving enables and all-at-once limits the connecting-separating with community as familiar-unfamiliar patterns arise with intensity.

Illustration of Driving

Jane, a woman who has been homeless, considers herself a community activist who focuses on helping people who struggle with limited resources. Her activities include a position on a steering committee that addresses the health issues identified by people with limited resources. In response to a long period of very hot and humid weather, and through her day-to-day dialogues with people who visited drop-in centers and food programs, Jane learned of many people who did not have any relief from the heat in their homes. They had no fans or air-conditioning. Jane made it her mission to find a way to get fans for these people. She began by contacting agencies that could identify people who needed fans. Then she compared prices and availability of fans in various stores. Jane presented the information to the steering committee, and, with her mission in mind, made a case for the steering committee to identify sources of funding and assist with writing a letter to prospective funding agencies. As the letter was being prepared, two members of the steering committee connected with possible funding sources, paving the way for Jane to move forward. The letter was quickly presented to an agency that approved the funding to go to a non-profit organization. Jane immediately contacted the local drop-in center and made arrangements for the money to be transferred to the center. Within 2 days the fans were purchased. In less than a week after Jane's initial contact with the steering committee, 70 fans were distributed.

Jane had recognized the urgency of the situation with the severe heat and humidity, and she was driven to find a way to provide fans for the people. She moved quickly, gathering relevant information and presenting the issue, with a solution, to the steering committee. The steering committee helped her to gain momentum by opening the most direct road to funding. Jane kept on going until she accomplished her mission. There was a constant quickening pace with brief periods of easing down, as Jane and the steering committee cocreated meaning approaching groups and removing barriers. This whole process was a coming together of people with diverse histories and a shared value priority for driving directly in moving-initiating community change.

Laddering

Laddering is climbing multidirectionally in planning and executing strategies in moving-initiating community change. Multidirectional laddering is not hierarchical. It is a labyrinthing process of moving all-at-once in many directions. In laddering, there is a pushing and all-at-once resisting in affirming multidirectional movement in conforming and not conforming with traditions, while fortifying the intent in face of the certainty-uncertainty of the looming potential disregard present with all community processes. The multidirectional movement in laddering is a way of connecting-separating that reveals and conceals the planning and executing of strategies, which both enables and limits accomplishing change with community. Planning and executing strategies for moving and initiating change are cocreated meanings of the moment, incarnating value priorities of community. These are lived in the process of laddering.

Illustration of Laddering

A regional consortium that focused on nursing workplace issues developed a plan to fund a nursing center to address the nursing shortage. The strategy consisted of a three-tiered approach to funding: monies from nursing licensing fees, private partnerships involving major healthcare organizations, and public funds. The public funds available were from a healthcare trust created by the state legislature. In order to obtain the funds, a law had to be enacted authorizing the disbursement of the funds for a nursing center. In planning the strategy with the community concerned with healthcare, it was determined that seeking the governor's support before initiating legislation would be essential to the process. All efforts would be in vain if the governor was not supportive. The first strategy was setting up a meeting with a member of the governor's staff, who offered advice on how to approach the governor to request her support. With the governor's support, the next strategy would be to gather support from key legislators and those concerned with healthcare throughout the state. Diverse value priorities of community were evident in cocreating the negotiating process. In the negotiating process, new meanings surfaced and, in going to the governor, the consortium made a multidirectional climb, strategically positioning itself by moving through a labyrinth-like process to the decision-making power. Then there were other directional moves to gain the support of the others so that eventually they could move again multidirectionally to climb with all barriers, to gain access to the desired funds in moving-initiating community change.

Boating

Boating is steering while navigating the calm-turbulence of shifting waves and winds, harnessing moments of buoyancy, yet always with the ambiguity inherent in moving-initiating community change. Navigating with community requires bridling the invigorating moments to coalesce resources when community is available to change. The availability arises as the cocreated meaning of the situation shifts. Steering is weaving with the familiar-unfamiliar in conforming–not conforming with valued traditions, while languaging new ways of connecting-separating with the diverse histories alive with community. There is certainty and uncertainty with shifting waves and winds that enable and limit movement, as community pushes and all-at-once resists in affirming intent in light of potential disregard. Ways of steering through calm-turbulent waves and winds reveal-conceal the value priorities of community.

Illustration of Boating

Lisa, 40 years old, embarked on her dream of pursuing doctoral studies. During the educational program, she was exposed to myriad worldviews and began to examine her beliefs. She chose a framework to guide her nursing practice that corresponded with her personal belief system. She believed that her views would be respected even though they were not consistent with the predominant paradigm of nursing. However, soon Lisa encountered challenges to her beliefs; though sometimes overt, most were subtle and often totally hidden from her. As she steered and navigated the deliberately planned course of study, she experienced turbulence. In cocreation of experiences with faculty and other students, she frequently was ridiculed for her belief system. Additional assignments were imposed, and she felt punished for not conforming to the values of a normative view of nursing. Lisa cocreated moments of refuge and support for her values by choosing to be with faculty and other students who espoused similar views, and by reading and attending conferences. Lisa, emerging as a scholar, steered toward graduation firmly connected to her value system, while at the same time drifting into new waters. There were moments of buoyancy as she met others with her view, but there was uncertainty as the waves and winds shifted. Navigating turbulent waves and wind with an all-at-once calmness cocreated both opportunities and restrictions for Lisa in moving-initiating community change.

Swimming

Swimming is gliding with diverse currents in keeping afloat with the sureness-unsureness of moving-initiating community change. Gliding is a rhythmical flowing, as community pushes and all-at-once resists in conforming and not conforming with the diverse currents of change. The diverse currents arise from personal histories, revealing and concealing the cocreated meanings present in connecting-separating. Community is enabled and limited by the imaged value priorities lived through languaging familiar and unfamiliar ways of keeping afloat.

Illustration of Swimming

Jean, a nurse educator and researcher, made careful preparations to conduct a research project in four different agencies with four diverse participant populations. She applied for federal funding for her research, since it would include traveling and handling a large amount of data. However, her grant application was not funded. Jean decided to go ahead with her plans to do research without federal funding.

Six months before her planned academic leave to conduct the research, Jean acquired Institutional Review Board (IRB) approval from all of the agencies involved except for one inner-city community health center, several hundred miles from her home, where the director for community care stated that IRB approval from Jean's university would be sufficient for her to have access to their population. Jean acquired IRB approval from her university and a letter from the director for community care stating she had met their requirements. The process of obtaining IRB approval from the various agencies required Jean to meet with personnel from the agencies, fill out individual agency IRB forms, and address all necessary recruitment protocols for each agency and participant group.

When the time came for Jean's academic leave, her plan was first to do the research at the inner-city community health center. She called the director of the center to let her know she was coming to the city and was ready to begin her data collection. Much to her dismay, she was informed that the director of community care was no longer employed by the center and the acting director stated she had never heard of Jean, nor had she been informed of her intended research. Jean was informed that she would be required to go through the center's new IRB even though she had the letter in hand stating otherwise. Jean traveled to the city to meet with the acting director, only to be told that she, too, was resigning and would be leaving the agency in 2 weeks. The acting director pledged to see that her IRB request was sent through the proper channels, but as Jean walked out of the agency with the forms, concern over how this request would be handled plagued her.

Jean decided she would go forward with the IRB request and rethink and reorganize her plan regarding what agency and what participant group would be her first focus for data gathering. Jean rhythmically flowed with the diverse currents of requirements of each agency, as she met IRB approvals to conduct her research. In spite of the resistance inherent in the absence of federal funding, she pushed ahead to implement the research. Jean treaded water to stay afloat as she encountered the new demands of the inner-city community center that were both enabling and limiting. Jean's way of viewing the situation changed with each new event. Jean flowed with the sureness-unsureness of changing agency personnel as she connected yet separated with them, determined to conform with the changing currents surrounding her research. Jean languaged the changing meaning of familiar and unfamiliar ways of keeping afloat in moving-initiating community change.

Submarining

Submarining is immersing in a high pressure enveloping at great depth with the shifting of what is known and not yet known explicitly in moving-initiating community change. High pressure situations are imaged valued possibles that reveal and conceal risks. With submarining, community is deeply engaged, meanings are shifting, and it is most important to take great care in moments of speaking–being silent and moving–being still. Community is enabled and limited with the shifting of the familiar with the unfamiliar in pushing-resisting, as conforming–not conforming escalates the uncertainties of potential surprise in connecting-separating.

Illustration of Submarining

Irene, a young woman who is living with cerebral palsy and muscular dystrophy, is wheelchair bound and has recently been diagnosed with breast cancer, for which she is currently undergoing treatment. She also has a variety of other challenges in her life that include carrying the pain of abuse, shattered trust, and the distancing of former close others. In the nurse-person process, there has been an immersion with all that Irene was, is, and will be. As community, Irene is the history she has been becoming, with all the predecessors, contemporaries, successors, ideas, and events that cocreate the meaning of her immediate moment. Irene says that living with cancer has sparked an intense enveloping examination of her life experiences, especially moments of suffering, in light of her hopes and dreams. She says that she feels a strong pressure to be heard for herself and others. She is committed to sharing her story for the benefit of all persons with disabilities. Irene and the nurse engage in intense nurse-person processes, sometimes three times a day, as the nurse lives true presence with her, bearing witness as she dwells with the familiar-unfamiliar of her becoming. Irene is submarining as she deeply envelopes with the situation in living the familiar-unfamiliar with shifting, escalating challenges that cocreate new meaning. She feels high pressure to conform with tradition, yet she risks disregard in calling others to her uniqueness. Irene sinks deeply as she lays bare her value priorities, revealing-concealing her imaged hopes and dreams. She moves to great depths in languaging her feelings as she chooses uncertain possibilities that may arise with the unexpected in moving-initiating community change.

Ballooning

Ballooning is drifting vigilantly with the pattern of the whole in a buoyant surgence-release, while shifting winds cocreate the unexpected in moving-initiating community change. In ballooning, community is cautiously watching the buoyant pushing-resisting of the ups and downs of the shifting winds, as imaged value priorities change and different meanings arise, cocreating a different reality, requiring new strategies. With ballooning, there is a revealing-concealing of community views in languaging the connecting and separating with the familiar-unfamiliar. Ballooning is both enabling and limiting as the certainty-uncertainty in vigilance is lived out in conforming and not conforming with tradition.

Illustration of Ballooning

Joanne is a 36-year-old vibrant mother of three young sons, who was working in a pain clinic when she was diagnosed with metastatic breast cancer. Even before her diagnosis, she had been nurturing her husband, Dave, in becoming a very involved parent. His development as a parent was especially important in light of Joanne's poor prognosis. The cocreated reality for the whole family shifted moment to moment as Joanne cared for the future of her family by working with Dave to select a nanny, a pediatrician, and appropriate schools. She even made arrangements with her older brother Bob to spend each Thursday with her three sons. All of the vigilant drifting with the pattern of the whole was especially important to Joanne as she contemplated the possible family trauma, especially to her youngest son, who was still in her womb at the start of her illness. The family members cautiously planned from a picture of the whole, as the imaged priorities shifted with the expected and unexpected. Anticipating her death, she supported all that she loved, while explicitly-tacitly knowing her boys would be fine. Six years have passed since her death, and there have been many buoyant surgence-releases in the lives of this young family. Bob adjusts his schedule to spend time with his nephews, and Ann, a pediatric oncology nurse, has joined the family as wife to Dave and mother to the children. The family illustrates how ballooning can continue as people cocreate different meanings with the shifting winds in moving-initiating community change.

Motorflying

Motorflying is propelling persistently with the gravity of weaving winds in all-at-once moving-initiating community change. With motorflying, the pushing-resisting with community is riveting in grave situations where achieving something of value is at risk. Motorflying is speeding with diverse imaged value priorities languaged amid the winds of disclosing-hiding, in connecting-separating with the familiar-unfamiliar. The meanings given to the propelling moments cocreate the reality that enhances and restricts movement. Motorflying is a community cocreation of persistently propelling with the certainty-uncertainty of choosing to conform and not conform with tradition.

Illustration of Motorflying

Sam, a 52-year-old man, lives with a spinal cord injury after a construction accident. Initially, after his prolonged hospitalization, he sought refuge in his house and would allow only a few select persons and his dog to interface with him as he lived a reclusive lifestyle. Gunter, an acquaintance of Sam's from the rehabilitation unit, persistently pursued Sam, inviting him to participate in new ventures that included kayaking, paragliding, and, eventually, wheelchair pulling. Sam relented, just to get Gunter off his back. Now Sam, whose meaning has changed, has become so involved in new ventures that he has organized sporting wheelchair events with basketball and polo competitors. He has persistently worked to arrange for local organizations to sponsor and purchase necessary equipment. He has accepted a position of authority to advocate for veterans living with disability, and he keeps in constant contact with legislators to address the needs of the disabled. He pushes hard with the resisting of self and others to achieve something he values as he weaves with the winds of change. He propels with adverse winds, affirming his being while risking with the chosen sports. Sam proudly states that he is enrolled in a course designed to teach skydiving—paraplegic style. With Sam's persistent propelling while understanding how it is to be living with a disability, he has cocreated a different reality that honors his individuality in moving-initiating community change.

Swinging

Swinging is soaring in undulating suspension with gusts of shifting winds in swingshifting to and fro in the bold leaping beyond of moving-initiating community change. In swingshifting, the undulating rhythms of community push and resist the familiar with the unfamiliar, while soaring with making a valued image possible, as meaning is cocreated with speaking–being silent and moving–being still. Swinging with the shifting winds of change cocreates a swingshift with the ways of connecting-separating change, enabling and all-at-once limiting a leaping beyond. The choices arising with swingshifting reveal-conceal the certainty-uncertainty of community change in light of conforming–not conforming with tradition.

Illustration of Swinging

Charles, a former U.S. marine, was in a diving accident 10 years ago. He injured his spinal cord and now describes himself as living with complete quadriplegia. In describing his life, Charles recalled what it was like in the days and months following his discharge from rehabilitation. He talked about going from being someone who was an active participant in social events, sporting events, and career-related activities, to someone who sat alone in his basement, in the dark, and felt sorry for himself. He slept a lot, rarely ate, and barely communicated with anyone. He described this as a devastating, horrible time in his life that went on for months and months. He said that sometime during that suspended mode, he began to imagine ways he could participate in things he liked to do, but in different ways. On occasion, Charles ventured out to try visiting his friends, or to participate in some group activity. There were often unanticipated barriers that led him to retreat by swinging back to the basement. This back and forth movement went on for several months until one day he accepted a job and began going out daily. Shortly thereafter, he joined wheelchair basketball and hockey teams, met a woman, and has since gotten married, and has two children—twin boys. Charles now devotes much of his time to helping others in situations similar to his. The sudden swingshift of change in Charles' life that came with his accident began a process of undulating suspension with shifting meanings. As he sat in his basement, alone, in the dark, he struggled with the was, is, and will-be of his situation. He experienced the shifting winds as he ventured out of the basement to experience his life in a different way. With each venture, the gusts of wind were challenging his choices and eventually he leapt beyond, cocreating a different life in moving-initiating community change.

Another Illustration of Swinging

The Health Action Model for Partnership in Community (HAMPIC) (Bunkers, Nelson, Leuning, Crane, & Josephson, 1999) began as a dream to bridge nursing theory to living the art in community. As the project director explored ideas with a core planning group, efforts were made to make this dream a reality. With much time and effort, significant support was obtained from area agencies and local foundations. A grant application was submitted to a major foundation. The group soared with excitement about the possibilities while waiting in undulating suspension. Despite great hope, the grant was not approved. Continued support from the area's funding agencies and foundations provided enough financial support to begin without the grant, and a HAMPIC nurse was hired. Discussions about the nursing practice model, creation of documentation tools, and the identification of sites unfolded in a to-and-fro movement that encompassed enormous risk-taking. HAMPIC was pioneering a new nursing presence that ultimately leapt beyond expectations.

Now, a steering committee meets quarterly to hear the voices of community. Members actively participate, cocreating a unique reality as they connect others to resources. Projects range from creating a medication dispensing system for street people, to linking a group of men from a third world country to higher education opportunities—all with very limited resources. A county- and city-funded service line has been added that provides nursing theory–guided advanced practice connections for families experiencing diverse health issues. Additional moving beyond is happening in nursing as nursing theory is studied and practiced with community. Students from both Germany and England have come to learn more about the practice model and its implementation. In a bold leaping beyond, the Board of Nursing in the area has studied and developed a decisioning model (Benedict et al., 2000; Vander Woude, 1998) that is based on the human becoming school of thought. Other boards of nursing are paying attention. Change has occurred amid shifting winds, gusts of wind have caught the attention of many, and there is a soaring with ideas and endless possibilities in moving-initiating community change.

Research Findings and Moving-Initiating Community Change

All of the processes (tunneling, driving, laddering, boating, swimming, submarining, ballooning, motorflying, and swinging) are lived all-at-once as ways of moving-initiating community change (individual or group). A research study that illuminates the meaning of moving-initiating community change is the one by Mitchell (1995) on restriction-freedom. Mitchell conducted a Parse research method (1987, 1998, 2001) study with 12 persons to discover the structure of the lived experience of restriction-freedom. The finding is "The lived experience of restriction-freedom is anticipating limitations with unencumbered self-direction, while yielding to change fortifies resolve for moving on" (Mitchell, 1995, p. 166). The participants in the study described ways they lived restriction-freedom. What they said is reflective of the idea of moving-initiating community change. They spoke of immersing, while yielding with change in moving on in new ways amid constraints. They forged directly, drifted, and climbed over obstacles, propelling with resolve to harness the moments of buoyancy to keep afloat in moving beyond with their envisioned possibles. They earthed and unearthed ideas in changing living patterns, while vigilantly flowing with and navigating the uncertain calm-turbulence of swingshifting to move barriers. These ideas connect the structure of restriction-freedom with the processes of moving-initiating change in living community.

Anchoring-Shifting Community Change

Anchoring-shifting is a cocreated paradoxical rhythm of community change. It is the persisting-diversifying that pushes-resists as community (individual or group) invents new meanings, knowing that all that was and will be is inextricably woven in the now. Anchoring the now with the remembered and the not-yet is an ever-changing process, since the remembered and the not-yet always arise afresh in the cocreated patterns of the now moment, as diversifying experiences shift the meaning of familiar-unfamiliar persons, ideas, objects, and events. The persisting-diversifying is what ongoing change means in light of the pattern of the whole. There is constancy recognized in the pattern of the whole and in the patterns of relating, yet everything is changing and no pattern is repeated. Juxtaposing change with pattern only has meaning with the all-at-once unfolding of both persistence and diversification. Persistence and diversification with community change relate to keeping some things and giving up others, revealing and concealing what is important while enabling and limiting the affirming of imaged possibles. The threads of constancy are intertwined with the diversity that comes with new experiences, cocreating the changing patterns of lived value priorities of community that are languaged in speech, silence, movement, and stillness. Community (all of the predecessors, contemporaries, and successors alive with the personal histories of an individual or group that is community) is enveloped in connecting-separating with the familiar-unfamiliar, as conforming to what was shifts in light of the certainty-uncertainty of change. The two major processes of anchoring-shifting community change are savoring-sacrificing and revering-liberating (see Table 4.2).

Table 4.2. DEFINITION AND PROCESSES OF ANCHORING-SHIFTING
COMMUNITY CHANGE

Anchoring-shifting is a cocreated paradoxical rhythm of community change.

Savoring-sacrificing is delighting in and all-at-once foregoing something of value.

Revering-liberating is honoring while all-at-once freeing.

Savoring-Sacrificing

Savoring-sacrificing is delighting in and all-at-once foregoing something of value in anchoring-shifting community change. Savoring is relishing ideas, objects, or events that are appealing to community, and these arise as threads of constancy. Sacrificing is giving up something originally delighted in and all-at-once taking on something else, the view of which has changed with new experiences. Meaning is cocreated anew as different value priorities surface, revealing and all-at-once concealing imaged possibles. Savoring-sacrificing is a way of connecting-separating with the familiar-unfamiliar in the certainty-uncertainty of conforming–not conforming. Savoring-sacrificing is an ongoing process of being enabled and limited in keeping while giving up. There is a pushing-resisting in the keeping and giving up that moves community beyond the moment in languaging imaged possibles.

Illustration of Savoring-Sacrificing

Jim, a 48-year-old investment banker with cardiomyopathy, retired early to spend more time with his family. He has a devoted wife and three children whom he has always attended to in special ways, but he also loved his work and was highly regarded by those with whom he worked. His talents brought him many financial and social rewards. He is community with the history of all his cocreated experiences. In retiring early, he savored the moments with family continuity and sacrificed his position, in anchoring-shifting community change.

Revering-Liberating

Revering-liberating is honoring while all-at-once freeing in anchoring-shifting community change. Revering is respecting others, ideas, objects, and events. Liberating is a buoyant freeing. Anchoring a pattern of honoring arises with weaving a shifting pattern of freeing as new experiences are lived with the opportunities and limitations of conforming and not conforming with tradition. Meanings change and are revealed and concealed as imaged values are languaged about honoring and freeing, in pushing-resisting with familiar-unfamiliar ways of connecting-separating. Revering-liberating is honoring and freeing with the pattern of the whole, incarnating the constant and the diverse in the changing value priorities of community.

Illustration of Revering-Liberating

Bill and Helen Jones have only one child, Allen. They attended to Allen with much care and concern throughout his life. Allen decided to move to a community several thousand miles from his parents to attend college. It was difficult for Bill and Helen to understand his decision since they were a close family. After many challenging moments and heated discussions, Bill and Helen decided to honor and respect Allen's choice to move to a distant city. They honored his choice, and, in seeing the pattern of the whole, Allen and his parents cocreated a liberating-revering pattern in anchoring-shifting community change.

Research Findings and Anchoring-Shifting Community Change

The processes (savoring-sacrificing and revering-liberating) are lived all-at-once as ways of anchoring-shifting community change (individual or group). A research study that sheds light on anchoring-shifting community change is the one by Pilkington (2000) on persisting while wanting to change. The extraction-synthesis of the 10 participants' descriptions led to the finding, the structure: "The lived experience of persisting while wanting to change is wavering in abiding with the burdensome-cherished as engaging-distancing with ameliorating intentions arises with anticipating the possibilities of the new" (p. 510). Persisting and changing all-at-once is reflective of savoring-sacrificing and revering-liberating. Participants in the study spoke of wavering between wanting to keep that which was cherished in their relationships, while wanting to give up the burdensome, and desiring protection from abuse as they engaged and distanced in making decisions. This is like savoring moments of worth, while sacrificing something of value. Personal decisions honoring priorities arise while freeing them all-at-once, as in the paradox revering-liberating. In living community there is always the anchoring force along with shifting patterns, as value priorities are made a reality and constancy and diversity prevail.

Pondering-Shaping Community Change

Pondering-shaping is a cocreated paradoxical rhythm of community change. It is contemplating while configuring. In living community, pondering what can be is present all-at-once with shaping what will be. Pondering-shaping arises in languaging imaged options with speech, silence, movement, and stillness for confirming–not confirming what community cherishes. It is contemplating reflectively and prereflectively the familiar-unfamiliar possibilities that all-at-once reveal and conceal the opportunities and restrictions of living with conforming and not conforming with tradition. Contemplating and all-at-once configuring is connecting-separating, cocreating new meaning in deep thought with others, ideas, objects, and events to carefully shapeshift change in a desired direction. With the certainties of shapeshifting, there is always the uncertainty of that which is not yet known explicitly in light of community aspirations and the pushing-resisting related to affirming change. The two major processes of pondering-shaping community change are considering-composing and dialoguing-listening (see Table 4.3).

Considering-Composing

Considering-composing is deeply contemplating while all-at-once birthing anew in pondering-shaping community change. Considering is ruminating or deliberating about others, ideas, objects, or events that are important for the moment. Birthing anew is creating or carving out the possibles. Imaged possibles cocreate new meanings that are languaged in composing ways of connecting-separating that reveal-conceal value priorities. The value priorities emerge with opportunities and limitations as certainty-uncertainty pushes-resists the considering-composing of the familiar-unfamiliar. Considering-composing is the structuring that arises with profound scrutinizing in pondering-shaping community change.

Illustration of Considering-Composing

Angela, a 25-year-old school teacher, is deciding whether to leave her position to return to school for doctoral education. She is pondering the possibilities and all-at-once shaping what will be for her. She is meeting with her social group and discussing her quality of life. Angela languages her vision, carefully considering the options, while composing a scenario with which she is comfortable. In speaking with her friends, Angela recognizes that she is enabled and limited with whatever decision she chooses. She pushes and resists affirming the possibles that are risky, as she is pulled to conform and not

---

Table 4.3. DEFINITION AND PROCESSES OF PONDERING-SHAPING COMMUNITY CHANGE

Pondering-shaping is a cocreated paradoxical rhythm of community change.

Considering-composing is deeply contemplating while all-at-once birthing anew.

Dialoguing-listening is unconditional witnessing with all-at-once speaking–being silent and moving–being still.

---

conform in living the certainty-uncertainty of moving with the familiar and unfamiliar in pondering-shaping community change.

Dialoguing-Listening

Dialoguing-listening is unconditional witnessing with all-at-once speaking–being silent and moving–being still in pondering-shaping community change. It is an emergent stream of meaning incarnating a unitary pattern of the whole. Dialoguing with community in pondering-shaping change arises with the discourse of the commingling of personal histories. Listening with pondering-shaping change arises with the astringent regard integral with coming to know something in depth while gaining an understanding, yet knowing that no understanding is absolute or complete. In dialoguing-listening there is a conveyance of meaning in witnessing. "Witnessing is beholding, an attending to with unconditional presence. It is dwelling with, incarnating availability" (Parse, 1999b, p. 1). The availability affirms the nonjudgmental presence alive in connecting-separating with the familiar-unfamiliar in the certainty-uncertainty of explicitly and tacitly unfolding the meanings of community in the moment and awakening to the mysteries of pondering-shaping community change.

Illustration of Dialoguing-Listening

Stephen is a 78-year-old gentleman who visited the nurse at the nursing center to discuss his latest experience with the healthcare system. During the nurse-person (community) process, the nurse bore witness to Stephen's expression of disquiet and hurt with the way he was treated by the healthcare system. He described being shifted from one doctor to another with no one offering any coordination of his care. The nurse listened with high regard for Stephen's concerns as he pushed and resisted affirming his value priorities, in light of the disregard he experienced. While he pushed to conform to an unfamiliar situation, he lived the certainty-uncertainty of connecting-separating. He spoke quietly with silences as he described moving with the system in moments of joy and sorrow, revealing and concealing who he was becoming in the enabling-limiting healthcare experience. The nurse, in dialoguing and listening, witnessed Stephen's situation, with an understanding that was neither absolute nor complete. Stephen's way changed as he illuminated meaning while speaking with the nurse. His understandings shifted the meanings in pondering-shaping community change.

Research Findings and Pondering-Shaping Community Change

The processes (considering-composing and dialoguing-listening) are lived all-at-once as ways of pondering-shaping community change (individual or group). Two Parse research method studies that shed light on pondering-shaping community change are on the lived experiences of considering tomorrow (Bunkers, 1998) and feeling understood (Jonas-Simpson, 2001). Bunkers (1998) studied the phenomenon of considering tomorrow with 10 homeless women. The finding is the structure, "Considering tomorrow is contemplating desired endeavors in longing for the cherished, while intimate alliances with isolating distance emerge, as resilient endurance surfaces amid disturbing unsureness" (Bunkers, 1998, p. 59). Participants in Bunkers' study spoke of thinking about what could be and what they desired would happen, in light of the unsureness of what might happen in shaping the not-yet. In pondering-shaping change with community, there is an imagining of the cherished with the unsureness of creating the desired aspirations of community. The pondering-shaping arose in considering-composing and in dialoguing-listening. The choices are cocreated and incarnate diverse perspectives.

Jonas-Simpson (2001) conducted a study with 10 participants on feeling understood. The finding of the study is the structure, "Feeling understood is an unburdening quietude with triumphant bliss arising with the attentive reverence of nurturing engagements, while fortifying integrity emerges amid potential disregard" (p. 92). The participants in this study spoke of their experiences of feeling understood as arising when people listen attentively and show respect for what is said and not said. The listening attentively confirmed the participants in their pushing-resisting of being with non-being. There is always the potential for the disregard of non-being during engagements with others, since understanding can never be absolute. This is true in all community situations where there is a desire to understand in shaping the not-yet. The finding of this study that sheds light on pondering-shaping change in living community relates to dialoguing-listening for understanding.

Illustration of Community Change: The Town Meeting

In this illustration each individual is community, and the group is community. Flyers were posted announcing a meeting in the community center of Tackley, a small village in Oxfordshire. The meeting had been initiated by members of the youth center, amid growing concerns over their personal safety when cycling around the village. They had tried to raise their concerns with local authorities and the police with no apparent success. In an effort to overcome their growing frustration, they visited the mayor's office and sought support for a meeting. They cited their concern about increasing traffic through the village, which placed their safety at risk when cycling. They also pointed out the danger to the environment and the quality of life. The mayor summoned his aides and agreed to immediately hold a village meeting to discuss these issues. The meeting was set for 6:00 P.M. on Tuesday.

Table 4.4. PERSONS AT THE MEETING AND THE HISTORIES OF WHO THEY ARE BECOMING

Youth Group	A group community. Members share common values regarding cycling and safety in the environment and bring with them their own personal histories and imaginings.
The Mayor	An individual community. He is a personal history with predecessors, contemporaries, and successors, a public figure with a vision.
The Youth Leader	An individual community. He is a personal history with predecessors, contemporaries, and successors, and brings his value priorities to his leadership position.
Jeff	An individual community. He is a personal history with predecessors, contemporaries, and successors. Jeff speaks on the issues of safety, environment, and quality of life.
Parents, Elderly Couple, and Whole Village	A group community. Members are personal histories with values and beliefs cocreated with predecessors, contemporaries, and successors. They give an example of an ever-changing process of becoming.

On that evening, the village hall was packed with young and old, families, and local business owners (see Table 4.4). A local youth leader chaired the meeting and called proceedings to order. The mayor was in attendance and listened intently to the dialogue as the villagers explored their common issues of concern. The youth leader drew on his skills of communication as certain sections of the village became entrenched with their values about traffic and village economy versus environment and young people's safety. Jeff, a 16-year-old boy who 3 months earlier, while delivering newspapers, had been knocked off his bicycle by a hit-and-run driver, stood to speak. He moved to the front of the hall and stated, in a very loud and determined voice, "I know not everyone agrees with restricting freedoms, especially those who drive cars, but I am before you to remind everyone of the consequences and risks to people's safety."

Following Jeff's statement, parents of three young cyclists moved to the front. These parents spoke of having met with young people to discuss the meeting and, as a result, learned just how many had had similar experiences, though not as serious as Jeff's. At this point an elderly couple were wheeled to the front and spoke of their growing fear when out in the village, because of the increasing village traffic and the lack of sensitivity to those in wheelchairs.

Jeff called upon all of the villagers to consider their future. He proposed that the village's main street be closed to traffic. In addition, the young people asked for bicycle trails to be created and for the main street to become a pedestrian-only area. The business owners spoke of the difficult economic issues that the changes would create. The plans would mean that much money would be needed to design the areas within the main street. Following discussion about this, a parking lot in the village center was added to the proposal to accommodate the concerns of business owners. There was a to-and-fro movement in connecting-separating as value priorities of community were revealed and concealed through languaging in speech, silence, movement, and stillness. The proposal was an imagined possible enabling-limiting the familiar and unfamiliar ways of pushing-resisting that arose in the discussions to affirm certain values in light of potential disregard. There was certainty and uncertainty, since creating the plan was a way of not conforming with the was, but was conforming with the new desires of community as group in moving-initiating change. There was anchoring-shifting, as the traditional values were honored with some changes that showed regard for the cocreated new value priorities. The entire process was a pondering of what was and what could be, all-at-once shaping the possibles of the unfolding proposal.

To the mayor's surprise, after much discussion the whole audience supported the proposal. The business owners were satisfied with plans to organize parking close to the village center, and all others were also satisfied with the plans for safety.

The community change arose at the town meeting as cocreated meanings surfaced a new reality ultimately agreed upon by all. The rhythmical patterns flowed, evenly and unevenly, as members of the village shared their concerns. The community pressed to move beyond, carving out a proposal for change that arose with pondering and shaping, as moving some barriers created new ones, and anchoring in the remembered shifted with the possibles (see Table 4.5).

Summary

The ways of living community change, as described in this chapter, illuminate structuring meaning multidimensionally, cocreating paradoxical rhythms, and cotranscending with the possibles. Community (individual and group) lives the explicit-tacit knowing of imaging in languaging with speech, silence, movement, and stillness in confirming value priorities. In living, community reveals-conceals what is important and is enabled and at-once limited with ways of connecting-separating. Community is pushing-resisting in powering originating to conform or not, even with the certainty-uncertainty that is present with all risking in transforming the familiar-unfamiliar.

Table 4.5. THE PROCESSES OF COMMUNITY CHANGE AS LIVED

Moving-Initiating Community Change

Tunneling	The youth's exposing the issue of safety was a deliberate unearthing of a safety and environmental issue. The earthing of tunneling was manifested when local authority figures did not respond to the issue. The values of both were manifested. Tunneling was also manifested when the villagers explored common issues of concern and unearthed what the situation was regarding safety and the environment. Unearthing was also shown in the business owners' concerns for economic survival.
Laddering	The youth climbed multidirectionally by going to the mayor and then bringing the issues back to the village and local authorities by planning and executing a town meeting.
Driving	The mayor forged with intense acceleration as he summoned his aides and set a meeting for 6:00 P.M. on Tuesday for cocreating changing patterns concerning safety and the environment.
Boating	The youth leader steered the discussion in turbulent waters (the entrenched villagers) while navigating for continuing the discussion of safety and the environment. The calmness of the youth leader steered community through the shifting waters of ambiguity, harnessing moments of buoyancy that occurred as people were heard.
Swimming	Jeff glided with the uncertainties of the diverse currents of the discussion by sharing his own personal story of being hit by a car. He kept his safety issue afloat as the village group continued discussions in a conforming–not-conforming manner of raising diverse opinions of safety and economics.
Motorflying	The three parents persistently propelled the issue forward, weaving the gravity of Jeff's situation with the other young people's experiences. The gravity was experienced by the entrenched villagers and the business owners. The leader, the youth group, the elders, the business owners—all were persistently propelling.

Table 4.5 (continued)

Submarining	The whole situation was submarining, a deep immersion in a situation where risking disregard was a challenge. The elderly couple in wheelchairs immersed with the other villagers in the high pressure of greater depth of understanding, shifting the familiar-unfamiliar safety-environmental issues of the village.
Ballooning	The mayor drifted vigilantly with the pattern of the whole by appointing a facilitator, creating a buoyant surgence-release while observing the shifting winds of opinion. He drifted as the villagers talked of possibilities. The unexpected surfaced in the agreement to move on with the proposal.
Swinging	The youth leader put forth the safety proposal in undulating suspension as the villagers considered a bold leaping beyond. A to-and-fro movement occurred as the business owners questioned the economics of the proposal and the parents and elders raised issues of safety and concern. Swingshifting occurred as the entire village agreed to the proposal. This was a bold leaping beyond in the moving-initiating of community change.

Anchoring-Shifting Community Change

Savoring-Sacrificing	All participants savored the view of safety while sacrificing some conveniences.
Revering-Liberating	Participants revered and honored the village residents, and, in order to promote the viability of the village, they accepted some freeing experiences.

Pondering-Shaping Community Change

Considering-Composing	Community contemplated the possibles about common concerns and differences and, while doing so, composed the proposal.
Dialoguing-Listening	Community dialogued and listened and shared concerns from various perspectives. Ultimately all agreed to change, bearing witness to each other.

The three concepts of community change (moving-initiating, anchoring-shifting, pondering-shaping), articulating the human becoming beliefs, invite different ways of being with people. This unitary view of community as indivisible, unpredictable, and ever-changing offers a new lens through which to view the human-universe mutual process. Community is boundaryless, a mystery defying standardization. Understanding community from a human becoming perspective arises with (a) knowing that removing barriers in conforming or not conforming to tradition creates other barriers; (b) knowing that while the shifting tides of change are ever present, there is an anchoring with the remembered that cocreates patterns anew, thus there is constancy with diversity; and (c) knowing that just imagining the will-be already creates the possibles.

The following tenets explicate the human becoming view of community as a oneness of human-universe connectedness incarnating beliefs and values:

- The individual is community.

- The group is community.

- Community bears witness–does not bear witness in unfolding meanings of the moment.

- Nurse-community process focuses on the hopes, dreams, desires, and intentions of community, one person or many.

- Nurse-community process is guided by community value priorities.

- Nurses are with community in digging, forging, climbing, steering, gliding, immersing, drifting, propelling, and soaring, as ways of moving-initiating community change.

- Nurses are with community in the persisting-diversifying of changing value priorities as the savoring-sacrificing and revering-liberating of anchoring-shifting community change unfolds with the changing patterns of preference.

- Nurses are with community in considering-composing and dialoguing-listening as ways of pondering-shaping community change.

References

Benedict, L. L., Bunkers, S. S., Damgaard, G. A., Duffy, C. E., Hohman, M. L., & Vander Woude, D. L. (2000). The South Dakota Board of Nursing theory-based regulatory decisioning model. *Nursing Science Quarterly, 13,* 167–171.

Bunkers, S. S. (1998). Considering tomorrow: Parse's theory-guided research. *Nursing Science Quarterly, 11,* 56–63.

Bunkers, S. S., Nelson, M., Leuning, C., Crane, J., & Josephson, D. (1999). The health action model: Academia's partnership with the community. In E. Cohen & V. De Back (Eds.), *The outcomes mandate: Case management in health care today* (pp. 92–100). St. Louis: Mosby.

Jonas-Simpson, C. M. (2001). Feeling understood: A melody of human becoming. *Nursing Science Quarterly, 14,* 222–230.

Mitchell, G. J. (1995). The lived experience of restriction-freedom in later life. In R. R. Parse (Ed.), *Illuminations: The human becoming theory in practice and research* (pp. 159–195). New York: National League for Nursing Press.

Parse, R. R. (1981). *Man-living-health: A theory of nursing.* New York: Wiley.

Parse, R. R. (1987). *Nursing science: Major paradigms, theories, and critiques.* Philadelphia: Saunders.

Parse, R. R. (1998). *The human becoming school of thought: A perspective for nurses and other health professionals.* Thousand Oaks, CA: Sage.

Parse, R. R. (1999a). Community: An alternative view. *Nursing Science Quarterly, 12,* 119–124.

Parse, R. R. (1999b). Witnessing as true presence. *Illuminations: Newsletter for the International Consortium of Parse Scholars, 8*(3), 1.

Parse, R. R. (2001). *Qualitative inquiry: The path of sciencing.* Sudbury, MA: Jones and Bartlett.

Parse, R. R. (2002). Transforming healthcare with a unitary view of the human. *Nursing Science Quarterly, 15,* 46–50.

Pilkington, F. B. (2000). Persisting while wanting to change: Women's lived experiences. *Health Care for Women International, 21*(6), 501–516.

Vander Woude, D. (1998). Nursing theory-based regulatory decisioning model in South Dakota. *Issues, 19*(3), 14.

CHAPTER 5

HUMAN BECOMING COMMUNITY CHANGE CONCEPTS IN AN ACADEMIC NURSING PRACTICE SETTING

WILLIAM K. CODY

The Charlotte Rainbow PRISM Model of community health nursing services delivery was synthesized from the philosophical underpinnings and key ideas of the human becoming school of thought originated by Rosemarie Rizzo Parse (1981, 1998), tenets of traditional community-based and community health nursing (Zotti, Brown, & Stotts, 1996), and nursing experiences in community-based service. The model has emerged from the faculty practice and community-based nursing service-learning projects of the Family and Community Nursing Department at the University of North Carolina at Charlotte. The major project, the Nursing Center for Health Promotion, a nurse-managed free clinic, serves the residents of a shelter for homeless women and children. The nursing center, though modest in size and scope, meets the definition of an academic nursing center in that it serves as a site for nursing education (undergraduate and graduate), nursing service (logging over 6,000 visits a year), faculty practice (community health nursing and family practice nursing), and research and scholarship. The stated mission of the Nursing Center for Health Promotion is to improve healthcare delivery for women and children who are homeless; to provide nursing services with sensitivity to diverse socioeconomic, cultural, and situational factors; and to foster diversity in knowledge and experience among faculty and students.

PRISM is an acronym for Presence, Respect, Information, Services, and Movement. The term *Rainbow* was added to express explicitly the faculty and staff's commitment to respect for human diversity. The logo for the model is shown in Figure 5.1. The purpose of this chapter is to explore interpretations of nursing practice situations in the Nursing Center for Health Promotion, where practice is guided by the PRISM model, in light of Parse's human becoming community concepts and processes as presented in this book. The development of the model pre-dated the introduction of Parse's new community concepts and processes, but situations and activities in the nursing center can be reflectively interpreted in light of the emergent concepts.

The essentials of the Charlotte Rainbow PRISM Model are as follows. Nurses are *present* with community. This means actually being there face-to-face, paying attention, being reliable, *being with* community in spirit and thought as well as immediate action, and staying with the community through major changes over time. Nurses *respect* community and the people who comprise it, profoundly, consistently without exception, and demonstrably. This means that it is the community members' visions of what is, what will be, and what might be, and their values and hopes and dreams that drive the providers' agenda as service providers. Nurses *seek information first,* and they listen, acknowledging the clients' freedom to make personal health-related choices. Then the nurses *make information available* to community, specifically *the information that the clients say they want and need* to support informed decision-making and self-sufficiency in healthcare. Nurses provide *services.* This means that community health nurses bring something tangible, useful, desirable, and meaningful, from the perspective of the client, into collaboration with community. Nurses encourage, support, and coparticipate in the *movement* of individuals and groups. This means that the nurses follow the lead of community members and change as the people change. The derivation of the model from the synthesis of its underpinnings from Parse's work and traditional community-based nursing is shown in Table 5.1.

Presence

Parse (1998) writes about *true presence* in the context of the human becoming school of thought as a "genuine, nonmechanical, nonroutinized attentiveness to others" (p. 99). She says it is "a special way of 'being with' in which the nurse is attentive to moment-to-moment changes in meaning as she or he bears witness to the person's or group's own living of value priorities" (p. 71). This definition provides key guidance to nurses implementing the Charlotte Rainbow PRISM Model. Parse further elaborates on her definition of true presence as witnessing:

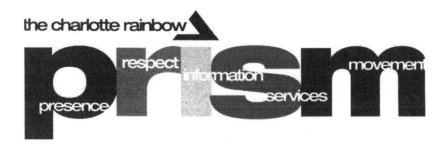

Figure 5.1. The Charlotte Rainbow PRISM Model logo. Copyright 2001 The University of North Carolina at Charlotte. Reprinted with permission.

Table 5.1. DERIVATION OF THE CHARLOTTE RAINBOW PRISM MODEL

PRISM Model	Human Becoming Theory	Tenets of Community-Based and Community Health Nursing	PRISM Model Definitions
Presence	True presence.	Working with people where they are, and offering help without judgment.	Presence is being with the community, face-to-face, paying attention, being reliable, being with community multidimensionally, and staying with community over time.
Respect	Profound respect for individual, family, and group values.	Respect for cultural diversity and individual differences.	Respect is profound veneration for human dignity, honored consistently, demonstrably, and without exception. This means it is community's values and hopes and dreams that determine the provider's activities.

Table 5.1 (continued)

PRISM Model	Human Becoming Theory	Tenets of Community-Based and Community Health Nursing	PRISM Model Definitions
Information	Focus on meanings, from the perspective of the person, family, or group.	Health education and dissemination of public health knowledge.	Information is of two kinds: information about clients, and information that clients want. The nurse listens first, last, and always, acknowledging clients' freedom and responsibility to make their own choices in life. Nurses make information available to clients that the clients say they want to support informed decision-making.
Services	Nursing as a human service guided by those we serve.	Population-based program planning based on needs assessment.	Services are helpful or useful acts on the part of nurses, directed toward clients, and are tangible, desirable, and meaningful from the perspective of the clients.
Movement	Transforming personal health by moving beyond the now moment.	Systemic change or behavior change.	Movement is change in a desired direction in the lives of individuals, families, and groups. Nurses encourage, support, and coparticipate in movement as determined by community. This means that the nurses follow the lead of the people served and change activities as people change.

Witnessing is beholding, an attending to with unconditional presence. It is a dwelling with incarnating availability. Witnessing is a non-intrusive gentle glimpsing in reaching beyond to honor the other as human dignity. The gentle glimpsing is a non-judgmental gaze embracing the other as a unique cocreation. Embracing is an unadorned intending acknowledging the significance of the other's choices; it is a standing with during a journey. Witnessing is living true presence. (Parse, 1999, p. 1)

Zotti et al. (1996), in defining community-based nursing (CBN) as distinct from community health nursing, write that CBN is "a philosophy of nursing that guides nursing care provided for individuals, families, and groups wherever they are, including where they live, work, play, or go to school" (p. 211). Blasser (2002) states essentially what every community health nursing instructor has taught students for years:

Nurses making home visits are guests in the client's home [home being wherever the client is].... We must remember to ask permission before we do something and be courteous and considerate to the homeowner or dweller. Anyone who has a "take charge" attitude will quickly get into a no-win situation. (p. 62)

From these disparate yet related views, the tenet of *presence* in the Charlotte Rainbow PRISM Model was synthesized and guides practice in the nursing center. Nurses are truly available to residents. Access is made as trouble-free as possible. The nursing center has an open-door policy and accommodates walk-in clients whenever it is open. It is located on the very grounds of a shelter and maintains open hours for the convenience of the women (3:00 to 7:00 P.M., Monday through Friday). Nurses and students are guided to intentionally convey availability and willingness to genuinely *be with*, to explore ideas and options and go with the person on the journey toward whatever, in any dimension of life, is valued by the woman or child in the moment.

Respect

The PRISM model's concept of *respect* refers to honoring human dignity and individuals' rights and responsibilities to choose from options in life. These ideas permeate Parse's writings, as seen in her descriptions of true presence (above). Gottschalk and Baker (2000), writing in the context of traditional community health nursing, suggest that equal, adequate healthcare for all "can only be achieved when the human rights of all, especially women, children, and those most marginalized and vulnerable, are promoted and protected"

(p. 3). Thus, traditional community health and community-based nursing emphasize respect for human rights and fundamental freedoms.

Rollo May (1981), whose views are similar to Parse's, has written that "freedom is essential to human dignity." He continues, "Human dignity is based upon freedom and freedom upon human dignity. One presupposes the other" (p. 9). Erich Loewy (1991), who writes from a more communitarian perspective, has stated:

> Respect denotes a measure of beneficence, an active interest in the welfare of others, and it logically demands not only that we refrain from actively harming those who are the objects of respect but likewise that we see to it that such people at the very least have their minimal needs met. (p. 64)

The PRISM model's concept of respect, then, is one of profound veneration for human dignity, which is honored consistently, demonstrably, and without exception. The values, hopes, and dreams of the community and its constituents drive the nurses' agenda.

The values, hopes, and dreams that are in the foreground of experience for the homeless women and children we serve are often, though not always, oriented toward the fundamentals as the people view them, such as food, clothing, work for pay, housing, childcare, education, and healthcare. The concept of respect in the PRISM model, then, synthesized from works of Parse and others, connotes a respect for whole persons, their personal, family, and group priorities, whatever these may be, and a concern of the nurse to contribute (with persons' guidance) to their achieving their desires. The nurses and students at the nursing center are present unconditionally and bear witness to the reality of the women's and children's lives as they are lived. The witnessing is nonjudgmental and in an atmosphere of profound respect for persons' human dignity. Key staff and faculty model this way of being with clients, and the atmosphere is promoted throughout the shelter consistently.

A self-care station demonstrates our respect for the freedom of the women we serve. Adult residents can use the self-care station free of charge, to select from an array of over-the-counter medications and other supplies (available to persons with cash in any drugstore, no questions asked) so as to care for themselves and their children. No examination is required, and educational materials and teaching are always available if requested, but are never required. The women's abilities to care for themselves and their children in the ways of their choosing is respected, and assistance with basics is available and given upon request in a way that betokens profound respect for the women's human dignity and freedom.

Information

The concept of *information* comes into the PRISM model from community-based and community health nursing and is not a concept that Parse discusses per se. The synthesis of ideas here, then, occurs in the way information is considered and used in practice. The nurse working in the PRISM model with clients first *listens* and seeks information from the clients about their situation, their values, their plans, and their hopes. The nurse encourages dialogue and communication client-to-nurse, client-to-client, parent-to-child, child-to-parent, and client-to-provider. The nurse is not considered a repository of information that is to be dispensed to clients as it is adjudged by the nurse to be needed, but is rather an attentive listener seeking to understand the person's perspective and to accompany the person on his or her quest for ways to make hopes and dreams a reality. The nurse recognizes and honors differences among people in all life dimensions and seeks to know what the person is seeking, from the person's perspective. This means not jumping to conclusions, not moving into an intervention-focused mode, not pressuring oneself as a nurse to teach or tell. The goal is to hear the residents and to convey a readiness to coparticipate in a dialogue about their concerns.

As an academic nursing center, the Nursing Center for Health Promotion has as a part of its broad mission health education for clients, which is available from students. Guided by the PRISM model, students in such teaching-learning situations are taught to seek to learn from clients what information is wanted and what information is most helpful from the client's perspective. Faculty and staff are encouraged and supported to practice in the same manner.

This way of engaging in the teaching-learning process with clients is referred to within the model as *client-directed education*. Information is provided to clients in accord with their wishes, not according to a predetermined plan made by the nurse or student. This may include information about methods of disease prevention and health promotion, how to access healthcare and social services in the mainstream system, information about disease processes, medication and non-medicinal approaches to living with various disease processes, and information about other human service agencies to facilitate the client's choice of action in a given situation. Residents very often request assistance to access additional care providers, or to determine what care is needed and available. From the community-based and community health nursing traditions, this type of assistance in gaining access comprises a part of the broad mission of the nursing center. This way of engaging the pursuit of information about access to services with clients is referred to within the model as *client-directed healthcare* planning. Online computer capability in the nursing center facilitates access to information.

Services

Parse (1998) regards nursing as a human service that is guided by those we serve. The nurse is seen as a not-knowing stranger and a servant. These ideas are incorporated in the Charlotte Rainbow PRISM Model. The model also draws on an orientation toward service that is drawn from the community-based nursing tradition of direct services, including both wellness and illness care, and the community health nursing tradition of population-focused programming based on the desires and wishes of community. The latter traditions are congruent with the purposes, functions, and operating requirements of an academic nursing center, wherein a service-learning project must meet community desires demonstrably and provide substantive educational experiences for students in undergraduate and graduate programs leading to degrees and licensure in nursing with specific requirements for knowledge and practice in these areas. The people we serve obviously have influenced the orientation toward service represented in the PRISM model. The nursing center functioned for many years without an explicit model, but was always managed by nurse faculty who sought to offer the clients what they wanted in terms of services. It has been made abundantly clear over the years that the women who access the nursing center for help are seeking healthcare services that are tangible, practical, and immediate. Hence, a key attribute of the PRISM model is that a range of services is offered consistently, and the services offered are selected so as to be highly desirable and meaningful, from the perspective of the clients.

Services are offered in three distinct professional roles, each with its own scope of practice: that of the registered nurse (staff nurses and undergraduate students), the advanced practice registered nurse (faculty, family nurse practitioners, and graduate students), and the advanced practice community health nurse (community health nurse faculty and graduate students). *Direct care* services are offered within the registered nurse (RN) scope of practice, viewed as an independent, professional, community-based role, and within the advanced practice registered nurse (family nurse practitioner) scope of practice, where the nursing component of the role is emphasized in offering whole-person, family-focused care. Many health concerns of residents are worked through with clients independently within the RN scope of practice, an attribute of the nursing center's operation that contributes valuably to the nursing education component of its mission. Services are never construed as merely fix-it solutions to medical problems but, rather, are offered in a context that is focused on the whole person and the family. For example, an age-appropriate children's book is offered to every child who undergoes a physical examination in the nursing center. As another example, a gathering of women for discussion and mutual support, which meets biweekly, was organized by the author in response to a stated desire for such a group, and regularly serves 7 to 10 women per week. *Indirect care* services are construed largely as facilitating connections between clients and resources and are of two kinds, *client-directed resource location*, and *client-directed system navigation*. Client-directed resource location is assisting clients to locate services and other resources within the geographic region in accord with their desires, intentions, hopes, and dreams. Client-directed system navigation is assisting clients to connect with desired services and resources in the maze-like complexity of the larger healthcare system.

Movement

The concept of *movement* in the PRISM model reflects the influence of the philosophical perspective on living that is embedded in Parse's human becoming school of thought. It has been construed to correspond with ideas elucidated by Parse (1998) with regard to *cotranscending with the possibles* in the theory itself and the practice dimension of *mobilizing transcendence*. In the human becoming school of thought, the processes of change, innovation, and evolution, as experienced universally by humans, are characterized as human-universe cotranscendence, in the abstract, and, at a more concrete level, *moving beyond the now moment*. In traditional community-based and community health nursing, movement has been characterized as behavior change in the individual, or systemic change, at an organizational level (Anderson & McFarlane, 2000). The concept of movement in the PRISM model is change in a desired direction in the lives of individuals, families, and groups, which is accomplished by mobilizing resources toward a desired quality of life. The nurse encourages, supports, and coparticipates in this movement as delineated in the model. Nurses follow the lead of the people served, and change whenever the desires of the people change. For purposes of documenting what happens at the nursing center's service-learning activities, the movement concept in the model also serves categorically to represent client outcomes. Outcomes in this model are conceived differently. These include enhanced client satisfaction; less time wasted in vain pursuits of services elsewhere; early detection, diagnosis, and intervention; desirable cost-benefit ratio (about $20 per visit overall); enhanced capacity for self-care—all in a context in which clients are the leaders in their care, thereby honoring and enhancing human freedom.

The Charlotte Rainbow PRISM Model in Relation to Nurse-Community Process as Described by Parse

The development of the Charlotte Rainbow PRISM Model of course pre-dates the development of Parse's new community change concepts and processes and her full elucidation of the nurse-community process in earlier chapters of this book. In this section of this chapter, the dimensions of the nurse-community process as described by Parse are explored in relation to practice as guided by the Charlotte Rainbow PRISM Model. A brief outline of the comparison is contained in Table 5.2.

The values embedded in the PRISM model that are inspired by Parse's work include the focus on the hopes, dreams, desires, and intentions of the constituents. Nurses learn about these from community, that is, individuals and groups. Nurses form impressions about the hopes and desires of the larger group through activities in direct and indirect practice. It is clear to those who follow the model that the intent of the nurse to focus on and stay with the desires, hopes, and dreams of constituents is living a commitment to a value orientation and is essentially the same whether the community is one individual or many. For example, an individual woman (community) with a unique personal experience and perspective on her life may seek a safe and confidential environment for testing for the human immunodeficiency virus (HIV), which we can provide (through a collaborative arrangement with another agency). Indeed, it was the repeated requests of many women over time that led to the nursing center's initiation of collaboration with another agency to offer the HIV testing on a regular basis.

Conversely, many women over time made known their wish that there be a women's discussion and support group (community) in the evenings so that they could get together with other women interested in self-improvement to talk about their experiences and issues. The group was initiated based on the cumulative input of women asking about such a group on site over the years. Now the group meets regularly, and the group meeting can be offered as an option to those women who express such feelings as "I wish I had someone to talk to," or "I feel so unsupported out here on my own and no one understands what I'm going through." When such occasions arise, the nurse guided by the model will respond, "Who, or what kind of person or group, would you like to be able to share your experiences with?" and will follow up with the offer of the group meetings if the woman expresses interest in this kind of experience.

Many, many times, a woman will express thoughts and feelings, desires, hopes, and dreams, in dialogue with the nurse, that reveal priorities that would not normally fit with the obvious priorities of the medical establishment. Often a woman will choose not to take the time to pursue her own

Table 5.2. COMPARISON OF PARSE'S NURSE-COMMUNITY PROCESS DIMENSIONS AND THE CHARLOTTE RAINBOW PRISM MODEL

Parse's Nurse-Community Process	*The Charlotte Rainbow PRISM Model*
Nurse-community process focuses on the hopes, dreams, desires, and intentions of the constituents, even if community is one person.	Nursing practice with individuals, families, and groups focuses on their desires and intentions. We are present on site consistently over time as well as multidimensionally through our persistent concern. We acknowledge individual freedom to choose direction in life and do not seek to influence or change persons' choices.
Nurse-community process is guided by community value priorities.	Nursing practice is guided by community priorities with utmost respect for values. In addition, nursing practice accommodates the purposes and functions of an academic nursing center, integrating nursing education, faculty and student practice, and scholarship.
Nurses bear witness while community is digging under, forging directly, climbing multidirectionally, steering while navigating, rhythmically flowing, immersing, drifting, propelling, and soaring, as ways of moving-initiating change.	Nurses bear witness to desires, intentions, hopes, and dreams of community. Nurses both bear witness to, and assist with, the clients' activities in pursuing their desires, intentions, hopes, and dreams.
Nurses are with community in the persisting-diversifying of changing value priorities as the savoring-sacrificing and revering-liberating of anchoring-shifting unfolds with changing patterns of preference.	Nurses are with community as values and intentions change over time, and nurses offer their energies to contribute to the attainment of desired changes.
Nurses are with community in considering and all-at-once composing dialogues that bear witness with community aspirations in pondering-shaping change.	Nurses listen and dialogue as community ponders and shapes the future. Nurses ponder and shape resources at the nursing center to conform with community preferences.

healthcare because she prefers to spend her time pursuing healthcare for her children and maintaining a job, even if she has highly serious signs and symptoms, such as very high blood pressure or excessive menstrual bleeding, that she knows merit medical attention. The nursing center seeks to accompany and support women in their choices. For another example, cigarettes are a source of comfort to many of the women, even those with respiratory ailments, and yet it is rare for smoking cessation to arise as a priority among the homeless women. The nursing center does not offer smoking cessation classes or the like, in light of the fact that smoking cessation is not a strong value for most of the women at the shelter who smoke. Frequently a woman comes into the nursing center voicing a specific concern, such as *headaches*, and, upon discovering that the nurse offers a welcoming, nonjudgmental presence and is wholly concerned with the woman's own priorities, ends up discussing various other aspects of her life situation at length, divulging stories of interpersonal violence, or intergenerational family discord, or children removed from her custody, or relational difficulties, depression, or mental illness. On such occasions, the nurse moves with the flow of the woman's personal story and stays with the priorities on which the woman chooses to focus.

That the Nursing Center for Health Promotion is an academic nursing center means that its overall purposes and functions include an integration of service to people, educational experiences for students, faculty practice, and on-going scholarship. The nursing center serves in this capacity for a wide variety of faculty and students and is supported by a variety of traditional sources of grant funding that demand accountability in quantitative terms. All faculty and students are expected to perform in congruence with the Charlotte Rainbow PRISM Model, but all are not expected to learn and utilize Parse's (1981, 1998) human becoming theory in its pure form, which guides the nurse to move entirely with the intentions, desires, hopes, and dreams of persons served, moment to moment, without exception. Numerous activities of the nursing center are structured to fulfill the necessary functions of an academic nursing center that serves as a site for both undergraduate and graduate education. Students in the undergraduate course Nursing Care of the Child have as a learning objective to perform a developmental assessment on a child. Students in the graduate course Health Assessment have learning objectives that relate specifically to the standard medical exam that they will be expected to perform in physicians' offices in later practicum experiences and upon graduation. All faculty, staff, and students who work in the nursing center, even for one day, are given an orientation that includes an overview of the PRISM model and a brief explication of its five major concepts. It is further imparted to all faculty, staff, and students who work in the nursing center that it is an expectation that all care, both direct and indirect, will be carried out in a manner that is consistent with the PRISM model. Faculty, students, and staff who work in the nursing center for extended periods of time are expected to attend periodic seminars on the model led by the author.

The lived experience of bearing witness characterizes the very core of practice guided by Parse's theory. The author and the long-time clinic manager are veteran *Parse nurses* who live the values and the beliefs of the theory every day. A number of the other nurses and nursing students who have worked in the nursing center have attended the local chapter meetings of the International Consortium of Parse Scholars, or learned about Parse's theory in the graduate nursing theory course, or have been sufficiently intrigued to seek further information about the theory and about living its values and beliefs in practice. The notion of bearing witness in true presence as the very core of practice has not been wholly embraced by all who work in the nursing center, but all are made aware of its centrality through the orientation process, and the clinic manager, this author, and others model bearing witness in true presence as a way of being with community, that is, individuals or groups. The PRISM model offers those practicing in the nursing center an opportunity to appreciate the tremendously diverse patterns of living experienced by the women and children residing in the shelter, which Parse characterizes in this volume as *digging under, forging directly, climbing multidirectionally,* and so forth. A composite study of community using the nursing center as an example follows. The shelter is different from the nursing center and different rules are enforced. The shelter does not follow human becoming tenets. The story that follows is of Janet and her children, who are staying in the shelter and visiting the nursing center where the human becoming tenets are followed.

Janet and Her Children at the Shelter

Janet is a 24-year-old mother of three children, Joshua, 8, Maya, 5, and Sean, 3. While she and the children had been living with her mother in an adjacent state, Janet had become concerned for the welfare of her children due to the presence of a man she felt she could not trust in her mother's home. She suspected that her mother's boyfriend had behaved inappropriately with her children while they were in her mother's care. Her mother denied that this was possible and refused to ask the man to stay away from the home. Rather than risk her children's safety any longer, Janet brought them across the state line to the homeless shelter, arriving on a Friday afternoon, only to find herself with minimal to no resources for supporting herself or her children in this new situation. When asked about her hopes from her new temporary base in the shelter, she said she hoped to gain access to a range of social services, to get into transitional housing, to obtain job training, and eventually to find adequate housing in the community and support herself and her children on her own. She was not in touch with any of the children's fathers and did not wish to pursue child support through legal channels, not believing that any of the men would be willing and able to pay it.

In her previous situation, Janet had worked part time without benefits in a fast food restaurant, though she had hoped someday to pass the General

Educational Development (GED) test for high school equivalency and perhaps to enroll in cosmetology school. She had secured food stamps and Medicaid benefits for her children, and had been able to live modestly and to meet minimum needs until she found it necessary to move across the state line. Although she had ensured that her children were immunized, well fed and clothed, and had seen a doctor when needed, she had not sought healthcare for herself since Sean's birth 3 years previously. In her personal life, Janet was accustomed to being her own boss, routinely kept late hours, and often had a beer in the evening to calm her nerves.

While she was at her mother's home, either her mother or a sister living nearby would keep Janet's children to enable her to work outside the home or run errands, but, once at the shelter, she found that her three children would have to have complete physicals to be enrolled in the on-site daycare. Until they had completed their physicals, Janet would have to keep them with her. Sharing baby-sitting with other mothers in the shelter was not allowed. Curfew was 8:00 P.M. and *lights out* was at 9:00 P.M. After lights out, scattered women and children in the 50-bed dorm talked off and on throughout the night, and there was rarely a moment of real silence in the facility, day or night. Beds were required to be vacated at 5:30 A.M. and the dorms vacated by 7:30 A.M. Meals were served rapidly and only at certain hours, offering whatever food had been donated, with no food available at any other time. No food, not even bottled water, was allowed in the dorms. Janet was disturbed by this policy, as she had been living with a diagnosis of hypoglycemia for several years and often had spells of feeling faint and irritable with the fluctuations in her blood glucose. All adult residents were expected to perform at least one significant chore every day, such as cleaning the 150-seat dining hall after meals. Accomplishing her chore proved to be challenging as there was no provision for childcare while she was doing the chore. She had brought along Sean's stroller even though she had rarely used it in months, and she found herself increasingly keeping Sean in the stroller because there were few other choices aside from chasing after him continuously. She noticed several larger toddlers and preschoolers in strollers in the shelter and realized this was a common means of dealing with the situation.

After arriving at the shelter on a Friday afternoon, Janet spent the weekend gathering sketchy information about options from the other women in the shelter, learning the shelter routine, and caring for her three children continuously. It was hard to sort fact from rumor, and many stories about social services and healthcare systems in town, gleaned from various women, contradicted one another. On Monday morning Janet attempted to see a social worker and was given an appointment for Wednesday with minimal further advice or information. She was told that when she saw her social worker on Wednesday there was a chance she would get some bus passes and instructions about which agencies to contact, and that the social worker might make a few calls for her, and she was disappointed, frustrated, and worried that this was all she could expect. By then she was completely out of cash, except for a few dollars in food stamps. She had no cell phone, and the only phone available to residents in the shelter was the pay phone.

By Monday afternoon when the nursing center opened, Janet had a large and growing number of concerns and was beginning to think perhaps it would be wiser to move back to her mother's home than to remain in the shelter. When she first came into the nursing center, not knowing what she might expect there except that the other women's comments about it were generally positive, she stated only that her three children needed pre-daycare physicals.

The pre-daycare physicals were quickly arranged with the nurse practitioner, serving as a preceptor to a graduate nursing student who would actually examine the children. The nurse asked Janet if she would be comfortable if two undergraduate nursing students from the Nursing Care of the Child course cared for the children so that Janet and she could talk for while, and Janet agreed. In a private cubicle in the nursing center, the nurse invited Janet to share more about her situation: "How has it been for you, coming to the shelter?" Janet replied that it had been much harder than she expected, although she had believed she was strong enough to do whatever it took to get her children away from a bad environment. She said:

> Now I don't know. I'm beginning to think that I've moved too quickly, that I've given up too much and got us into a worse situation. I thought there would be more help here at the shelter than there is, and this is really rough. I didn't know the routine here would be so strict, that it would be so hard to sleep, that just getting a meal or getting a shower would be such an ordeal. It's rough on the kids, but they don't realize just how much trouble we're in, and I'm trying to protect them from realizing it. So it's especially rough on me, and if I don't get some relief from constantly having to be watching over these three kids I feel like I'm going to go insane!

The nurse let Janet know that the younger two children would be eligible to be enrolled in the shelter's daycare program the following day if the physicals showed no problems, and asked, "What will you do once you have some time free of the younger kids?" Janet said she would love to be able to go job-hunting, so as to get some cash as quickly as possible, but she knew that that would not be possible. Even unencumbered by constant care for the two younger children once they were in daycare, she would still have 8-year-old Joshua with her, and they actually had even more pressing needs than cash. She would turn her attention to getting social services in this new location, getting their Medicaid insurance transferred to this new state, and getting the older two children into the public schools. The nurse asked Janet how she prioritized these needs, and then offered information in that order as to how each goal could be pursued with the community (agency names, phone numbers, business hours, bus routes, rules and regulations, and so forth). The nurse also invited Janet to take a short break while the children were being cared for by the nursing students and offered her the use of the cubicle to relax for a few minutes with a sound machine playing her choice of a light rain, ocean waves, a summer night, and so forth. Janet immediately accepted, and she enjoyed a brief relaxing respite in the cubicle in the nursing center in the midst of the chaos. Before Janet left that evening with the children, the nurse gave her several bus passes to help her to pursue the resources she intended to seek. The nurse also reminded Janet that the nursing center was open every afternoon and evening from 3:00 to 7:00 and that she and her children were welcome to stop by anytime for any reason.

Over the next few weeks, Janet dropped into the nursing center, at least briefly, more evenings than not as she struggled to establish access to the services and resources that she wanted for her children and herself. Each time Janet dropped by, she was invited by the nurse to talk about whatever she wished, and the nurse listened and focused on Janet's priorities. Janet enrolled Joshua and Maya in school, and was placed in contact with a local agency dedicated to meeting the schooling requirements of homeless children, which augmented the family's school-related resources with information about the county school system, agency programs, and school supplies, and established communication with Joshua's and Maya's teachers. Sean was enrolled in daycare, and Janet was able to pursue her daily goals with hopes of getting the family on its feet. Her mother came to visit, and, although the meeting was tense, she left Janet with $50 cash to ease the hardships with which she and the children were living.

As the little family moved through the unfamiliar and uncomfortable routines of the days, many aspects of life at the shelter wore on Janet, and she took advantage of the attention offered her by the nurses in the nursing center to express her frustrations, disappointments, intentions, hopes, and dreams. Sorting fact from rumor, misinformation, and miscommunication continued to be a problem, in a context of seemingly intractable disinterest and disregard among many agency employees, and many forays into the world at-large to secure goods and services for her family came up empty. All one could do was retreat into the shelter for a day or two to rest, then venture out again.

Janet found living with 250 people in extremely close quarters to be far more challenging than she had imagined. A number of the women had little education, had basically lived on the streets for years, and had problems with drugs or even violent behaviors. Even though it was banned from the shelter, corporal punishment of the children by their mothers was common, and Janet saw that this was something the silent code among the women forbade reporting. The residential advisors who oversaw the dorms often abused their powers, ordered women and children around needlessly, and threatened a write up constantly. Headaches were so common among the women as to be almost ever-present, tempers were short, and the use of rationality to resolve conflicts was scarce; rather, it was authority or power that won out more often than not.

After a while, Janet met and became close to Catherine, another young single mother who resided at the shelter with her 6-year-old daughter, Mandy. Confidants, companions, mentors, and allies were extremely important in the shelter, and making a connection with Catherine strengthened Janet's resolve, bolstered her confidence, and called up her hope. Janet and Catherine shared knowledge and information about working the system and began surreptitiously to care for each other's children so that the other could run errands, make phone calls, or visit the nursing center. The three older children were able to share a pattern of daily living so that it became familiar, and Sean spent more time running and playing and less in the stroller. Janet and Catherine traded turns attending the evening group meeting at the center, one on Tuesday and one on Thursday. They even traded turns going out for a drink once in a great while, while in each case all four children remained behind with one mother looking after them, which offered a delightful break from the grinding routine. At first, Janet tried to abide by the ban on food in the dorms even though she had some very unpleasant nights, between the chatter and her symptoms of hypoglycemia, but then she noticed that a number of the women secretly brought water, bottled iced tea, candy bars, and other foodstuffs into the dorms, and she began to stash some food in her locker, which made the nights a little more bearable. Using the remaining food stamps gave her a sense of freedom. Janet's mother continued to visit occasionally and usually gave her at least $10 or $20 "to buy something for the kids."

With determination and effort, Janet was able to access some social service benefits and to begin the process of transferring the children's Medicaid insurance to their new state of residence. Then she focused intently on finding work and rapidly filled out numerous job applications. Toward the end of her second week at the shelter she was offered a position in food services, which came, unfortunately, without benefits or paid time off. The salary, however, would be sufficient to save toward the next step, her GED and further job training, while living rent-free at the shelter. In order to take the position, Janet was required to have a physical exam, which was of course offered free of charge in the nursing center.

During the previous 2 weeks they had worked with Janet the nurses had never pressed her to have a physical examination, nor had they been inquisitive about her private affairs or personal health beyond asking what her concerns were and what help she felt she needed. Janet had made it very clear that her priorities were the well-being of her children, the pursuit of a good job, and a secure home life for her family. Her history and physical exam revealed a number of areas in which Janet could use further services, such as hypoglycemia, a history of treatment for several sexually transmitted diseases (STDs) without the recommended follow-up, the fact that Janet had lost her eyeglasses several years before, and various other issues.

When the history and physical brought these issues to light, the nurse practitioner shared recommendations with Janet from standards of medical practice, and the nurse was attentively present with Janet as she explored her options. The nurse asked Janet, "Now that you have this information, what would you like to do about it?" Janet replied that maybe it was time that she turn her attention to herself, having dedicated the lion's share of her energy to her children for many years, and asked the nurse to help her find the appropriate resources to deal with her situation. The nurse offered to assist with client-directed health planning, client-directed resource location, and client-directed system navigation, and the dialogue continued with a focus on meeting Janet's long-deprioritized healthcare situation, the exploration of options, and the development of a plan for moving on. With up-to-date, fine-tuned information about local systems from the nurses, and their encouragement to pursue whatever she wished, Janet sought and eventually obtained the healthcare resources that she chose to pursue. With information about dietary habits in relation to hypoglycemia, Janet created her own modified daily eating plan. With assistance from the nursing center staff, she contacted the Lion's Club, which provides eyeglasses to low-income people free of charge, and obtained her eyeglasses. She followed up on her past history of STDs through the local health department and found that the situations had been resolved with the previous treatment.

As time passed, Janet and Catherine became closer, and, since they were both working but constantly needed help to care for the children, they began to discuss someday obtaining housing together. Toward this end, they both began to save their take-home pay more intently. Helping each other to watch the children, they were each able to work more hours. Eventually they left the shelter and moved in together with their children. Janet left the shelter telling the nurses that she had already obtained all the information she needed to begin planning to enroll in cosmetology school. Janet's story is shown in relation to Parse's community concepts in Table 5.3.

Moving-initiating change is described by Parse as moving barriers while creating new ones, discarding and creating all-at-once, making reality of the valued visions of community. Janet chose to leave her mother's home to remove her children from suspected abuse. Moving to the shelter with the children accomplished the major goal of removing the children from an unsafe situation but also brought the family (community) face-to-face with many new challenges and obstacles, as described earlier. Parse described nine processes of moving-initiating community change: tunneling, driving, laddering, boating, swimming, submarining, ballooning, motorflying, and swinging. In Table 5.3 elements of Janet's story are interpreted in light of the moving-initiating community change concepts and processes.

Anchoring-shifting change is described by Parse as anchoring the now with the remembered and the not-yet; it is the persisting-diversifying rhythm of change in connection with the evolution of the familiar-unfamiliar among the persons, ideas, and events of one's life. Janet remained committed to caring for her children and maintaining family closeness although she and her mother were somewhat estranged. Though their relationship changed irreversibly, her mother visited and was welcomed and tried to help out with

Table 5.3. ILLUSTRATION OF THE CORRESPONDENCE BETWEEN JANET'S STORY AND THE HUMAN BECOMING COMMUNITY CONCEPTS

Janet chose to leave her mother's home to remove her children from suspected abuse. Moving to the shelter with the children entailed an array of new challenges and obstacles, including many restrictive rules and the absence of social service benefits. Janet's displeasure with her mother's attitude and her assessment of her children's endangerment meant for her that getting out was important enough to accept the hardships of the new situation.	Moving-initiating—a cocreated paradoxical rhythm of community change. Community moves and initiates constraints all-at-once.
Janet, like all the women at the shelter, shared the information that she chose with the staff in the shelter and the nurses in the nursing center, and kept other information to herself. She hid food to avoid abuse of power.	Tunneling—digging under; piercing the depths; earthing and unearthing.
Upon finding herself in an unpleasant situation with her three children, Janet forged ahead in making changes, moving the family across the state line, rapidly accessing social service benefits, daycare, and schools, and getting a job.	Driving—forging directly; an intense quickening pace with an easing down.
Janet surmounted many obstacles to pursue her hopes and dreams. She tracked down information, found work, obtained social services, arranged healthcare for her children and herself, and kept planning to complete the GED and pursue further education to secure a better income in the future.	Laddering—climbing multi-directionally in planning and executing strategies.
Janet steered quietly through the often-chaotic daily activities at the shelter and the sometimes unpleasant interactions with others while seeking to protect her children from the harshness of the situation and to minimize conflicts with the other women.	Boating—steering while navigating the calm-turbulence of shifting waves and winds.
Janet allowed the flow of activities in the shelter and in pursuit of social services to carry her along when there was nothing else she could do but tread water and wait.	Swimming—gliding with diverse currents in keeping afloat.

Table 5.3 (continued)

Like many women in the shelter, Janet focused intently on the priorities she held out for herself and her family in the high-pressure environment of the shelter. She used the time and the less-than-optimal assistance available to plan for the future and arrange matters as well as she could.	Submarining—immersing in a high pressure enveloping at great depth with the shifting of what is known and not yet known.
Janet "lay low" in the shelter, drifting with the sometimes unpleasant flow of the environment so as to not make unwelcome waves. Although the rules were oppressive and the interpersonal challenges were many, she didn't protest or rebel, and eventually she met Catherine, with whom she could better "work the system" surreptitiously to pattern her life more to her liking while in the shelter.	Ballooning—drifting vigilantly with the pattern of the whole in a buoyant surgence-release, while shifting winds cocreate the unexpected.
After years of living with her mother, working part-time, and enjoying leisure time, Janet worked rapidly to transform the situation that she found herself in, working many hours and strategizing and collaborating with Catherine and the nurses in her off hours. She was propelling herself toward success amid the swirling winds of an uncertain place in society and chaos in the shelter.	Motorflying—propelling persistently with the gravity of weaving winds.
Although many forays into the world at-large were unproductive in her attempts to meet the needs of her family, after a brief respite in the shelter Janet would marshal her energies to venture back out again in pursuit of a better life.	Swinging—soaring in undulating suspension, swingshifting in the bold leap forward.
Janet remained committed to caring for her three children and maintaining family closeness although she and her mother were somewhat estranged. Though their relationship changed, her mother visited and tried to help out with money. Janet found in Catherine a new source of comfort and support, and the two families chose to move forward together.	Anchoring-shifting—a cocreated paradoxical rhythm of community change. Community invents the new, anchoring the now with the remembered and the not-yet; diversifying experiences shift meanings.

Table 5.3 (continued)

Janet and Catherine moved with the rhythms of giving up much of their adult social life to abide by shelter rules, while also at times indulging in the secret pleasure of helping each other to slip out for a brief time away from the children and have a drink.	Savoring-sacrificing—delighting in and all-at-once forgoing something of value.
Janet respected her mother and did not wish to hurt her, but she knew she had to leave and take the children. Her mother respected her concerns but wished to continue with her boyfriend, and so they were free to live together after Janet left. Janet and Catherine ostensibly abided by all shelter rules and demonstrated respect to the staff while also taking steps to live at times in chosen ways that violated the stated code of the shelter.	Revering-liberating—honoring while all-at-once freeing; honoring what is while freely coparticipating in cocreating what is not yet.
Janet reflected on her wishes, priorities, and dreams, sometimes in the presence of the nurse, and she chose from options how to be in her new situation and what course of action to take.	Pondering-shaping—a cocreated paradoxical rhythm of community change. Community contemplates while configuring.
Janet shared her story at various times with her mother, with the nurses, with the social workers and staff in the shelter, with other agency workers, and with the women in the shelter. Her telling and their responses shaped possibilities of what could come of the interactions.	Considering-composing— deeply contemplating while all-at-once birthing anew.
Janet listened carefully to her mother's response to her concerns about abuse, to the other women in order to learn about survival in the shelter, and to nurses and social service representatives when trying to access resources. The nurses listened carefully to Janet as she described her intentions, priorities, hopes, and dreams, so as to offer what services and information she wanted. Her telling and their responses shaped possibilities of what could come of the interactions.	Dialoguing-listening— unconditional witnessing with all-at-once speaking–being silent and moving–being still.

money. Janet, while laboring to sustain her own family, also found a new source of comfort and support in connecting with Catherine and Mandy, and eventually the two families chose to move forward together. Parse described two concepts within anchoring-shifting: savoring-sacrificing and revering-liberating. In Table 5.3 elements of Janet's story are interpreted in light of the concept anchoring-shifting community change and its processes.

Pondering-shaping change is described by Parse as contemplating while configuring anew, contemplating what can be while configuring what will be. Janet reflected on her wishes, priorities, and dreams, oftentimes in the presence of the nurse, as she chose from options how to be in her new situation and what course of action to take. Parse described two processes of pondering-shaping: considering-composing and dialoguing-listening. In Table 5.3 elements of Janet's story are interpreted in light of the concept pondering-shaping community change and its processes.

Conclusions

The author in this chapter offered interpretations of nursing practice situations in the Nursing Center for Health Promotion, where practice is guided by the Charlotte Rainbow PRISM Model, in light of Parse's human becoming community change concepts and processes as presented in this book. Further reflection will undoubtedly contribute to the ongoing process of refining and improving the PRISM model. Parse's creative conceptualization of community change concepts from a human becoming perspective is a major and original contribution to the literature, which offers to nurses myriad opportunities to challenge the status quo with innovative nursing practice models inspired and guided by the human becoming school of thought.

References

Anderson, E. T., & McFarlane, J. (2000). *Community as partner: Theory and practice in nursing* (3rd ed.). Philadelphia: Lippincott.

Blasser, C. T. (2002). Preparing students for home visits. In G. M. Redmond & J. M. Sorrell, *Community-based nursing curriculum: A faculty guide* (pp. 53–69). Philadelphia: Davis.

Gottschalk, J., & Baker, S. S. (2000). Primary health care. In E. T. Anderson & J. McFarlane, *Community as partner: Theory and practice in nursing* (3rd ed.) (pp. 3–25). Philadelphia: Lippincott.

Loewy, E. (1991). *Suffering and the beneficent community: Beyond libertarianism*. Albany: State University of New York Press.

May, R. (1981). *Freedom and destiny*. New York: Norton.

Parse, R. R. (1981). *Man-living-health: A theory of nursing.* New York: Wiley.

Parse, R. R. (1998). *The human becoming school of thought: A perspective for nurses and other health professionals.* Thousand Oaks, CA: Sage.

Parse, R. R. (1999). Witnessing as true presence. *Illuminations: Newsletter of the International Consortium of Parse Scholars, 8*(3), 1.

Zotti, M. E., Brown, P., & Stotts, R. C. (1996). Community-based nursing versus community health nursing: What does it all mean? *Nursing Outlook, 44,* 211–217.

CHAPTER 6

COMMUNITY: AN EMERGING MOSAIC OF HUMAN BECOMING

SANDRA SCHMIDT BUNKERS

On a June night in 2001, at St. John's University in Collegeville, Minnesota, at the Institute for Ecumenical and Cultural Research, I was standing on a small grassy hill with several other scientists, looking through a high-powered telescope pointed toward the stars. Being coached by an astronomer, I was told to look through the telescope in a certain direction. He stated, "You will see another universe." And, I did! The astronomer went on to say, "That brilliant constellation you see is how we look from that vantage point, over 1 million light years away."

Our St. John's community of scholars was composed of a variety of persons from scientific, theological, and philosophical backgrounds, including three philosophers from Moscow and St. Petersburg, Russia. This international community of scholars was gathered to discuss ideas regarding the interface of religion and science. Seeing the other universe brought to awareness the need to look beyond our individual worlds and even our collective world in seeking to understand the purposes that religion and science play in the mystery of human becoming. It keenly brought to my attention the interconnectedness of all things. I mindfully reflected on the fact that community consists of *all that is*. As Parse (2003) writes, "Community ... is a oneness of human-universe connectedness incarnating beliefs and values" (p. xi). Community is a mosaic of human becoming, a configuration of beliefs, values, choices, and personal histories with predecessors, contemporaries, and successors all-at-once in mutual process with all that is.

This unitary view of community calls for a foundational shift in how nursing perceives community in addressing quality of life for humankind. In this book Parse sets forth a new view of community from the human becoming perspective. Presented in this chapter is an exploration of community nursing using the human becoming community change concepts created by Parse. First, a glimpse of the present is discussed.

Several conceptualizations of community nursing models have attempted to synthesize public health science, community health nursing concepts, and nursing theory (Davis, 2000; Rafael, 2000; Raphael et al., 1999). However, these theoretical models continue to describe community as a place one goes to, instead of a process one engages in (Bunkers, Michaels, & Ethridge, 1997; Parse, 1999). The American Nurses Association (ANA) *Scope and Standards of Public Health Nursing Practice* (1999) also support the conceptualization of community as a place one goes to work with groups, aggregates, and special populations (see Table 6.1). Both the community models mentioned above and the ANA Standards of Public Health Nursing Practice are aligned with the totality paradigm in nursing (Parse, 1987).

As an alternative, a simultaneity paradigm nursing theory–guided community model, The Health Action Model for Partnership in Community (HAMPIC) (Bunkers, Nelson, Leuning, Crane, & Josephson, 1999), was developed in 1997 in Sioux Falls, South Dakota, to build on the conceptualization of community as process, and it is still in operation today. The health action model, based on Parse's (1981, 1998) human becoming school of thought, defines community as living in relationship (see Figure 6.1). This community nursing model focuses on the connections-disconnections existing with community. Nurses work with persons struggling with economic, social, and interpersonal difficulties in "creating personal health descriptions and health action plans" (Bunkers et al., 1999, p. 96). In creating health action plans the nurses work with community in exploring hopes and fears for changing patterns of health, thus changing the community's quality of life. Objectives of the health action model include (a) creating a nursing model to guide provision of health services for individuals and families experiencing disconnection from economic, social, and interpersonal resources; (b) utilizing the health action model to address health issues of *site* communities; (c) providing educational experiences for students in nursing and other health professions, focusing on understanding diversity and healthcare disparity; and (d) extending the health action model beyond the local area and sharing it as a prototype for healthcare in community regionally, nationally, and internationally (Bunkers et al., 1999).

The historical evolution of the health action model is manifested in Bunkers' (2002) identified processes for developing nursing theory–guided models. These are not linear in nature but are "ongoing mutual processes of envisioning what can be" (Bunkers, 2002, p. 174). Bunkers' processes of model development include *imaging the vision; engaging community; developing a conceptual framework; naming operational components; creating a documentation system;*

Table 6.1. STANDARDS OF PUBLIC HEALTH NURSING PRACTICE

Standards of Care

Standard I. Assessment

The public health nurse assesses the health status of populations using data, community resources identification, input from the population, and professional judgment.

Standard II. Diagnosis

The public health nurse analyzes collected assessment data and partners with the people to attach meaning to those data and determine opportunities and needs.

Standard III. Outcomes Identification

The public health nurse participates with other community partners to identify expected outcomes in the populations and their health status.

Standard IV. Planning

The public health nurse promotes and supports the development of programs, policies, and services that provide interventions that improve the health status of populations.

Standard V. Assurance: Action Component of the Nursing Process for Public Health Nursing

The public health nurse assures access and availability of programs, policies, resources, and services to the population.

Standard VI. Evaluation

The public health nurse evaluates the health status of the population.

Standards of Professional Performance

Standard I. Quality of Care

The public health nurse systematically evaluates the availability, accessibility, acceptability, quality, and effectiveness of nursing practice for the population.

Standard II. Performance Appraisal

The public health nurse evaluates his or her own nursing practice in relation to professional practice standards and relevant statutes and regulations.

Table 6.1 (continued)

Standard III. Education

The public health nurse acquires and maintains current knowledge and competency in public health nursing practice.

Standard IV. Collegiality

The public health nurse establishes collegial partnerships while interacting with healthcare practitioners and others, and contributes to the professional development of peers, colleagues, and others.

Standard V. Ethics

The public health nurse applies ethical standards in advocating for health and social policy, and delivery of public health programs to promote and preserve the health of the population.

Standard VI. Collaboration

The public health nurse collaborates with the representatives of the population and other health and human service professionals and organizations in providing for and promoting the health of the population.

Standard VII. Research

The public health nurse uses research findings in practice.

Standard VIII. Resource Utilization

The public health nurse considers safety, effectiveness, and cost in the planning and delivery of public health services when using available resources, to ensure the maximum possible health benefit to the population.

Adapted from American Nurses Association. (1999). *The Scope and Standards of Public Health Nursing Practice*. Washington, DC: American Nurses Publishing. Copyright 1999 American Nurses Publishing, American Nurses Foundation/American Nurses Association. Adapted with permission.

participating in teaching-learning processes; obtaining funding; conducting research; and *publishing the prototype.*

Imaging the vision involves conceptualizing the focus and purposes of the practice model, and inviting others to capture the vision. The focus of the health action model is quality of life from the community's perspective. Health is defined as human becoming (Parse, 1990), and community is understood as a process of living in relationship. An example of articulating the purposes of the model and inviting others to capture this vision can be seen in a newly developed program within the HAMPIC entitled The Dakota Network Project. A human becoming nurse works with nine community health

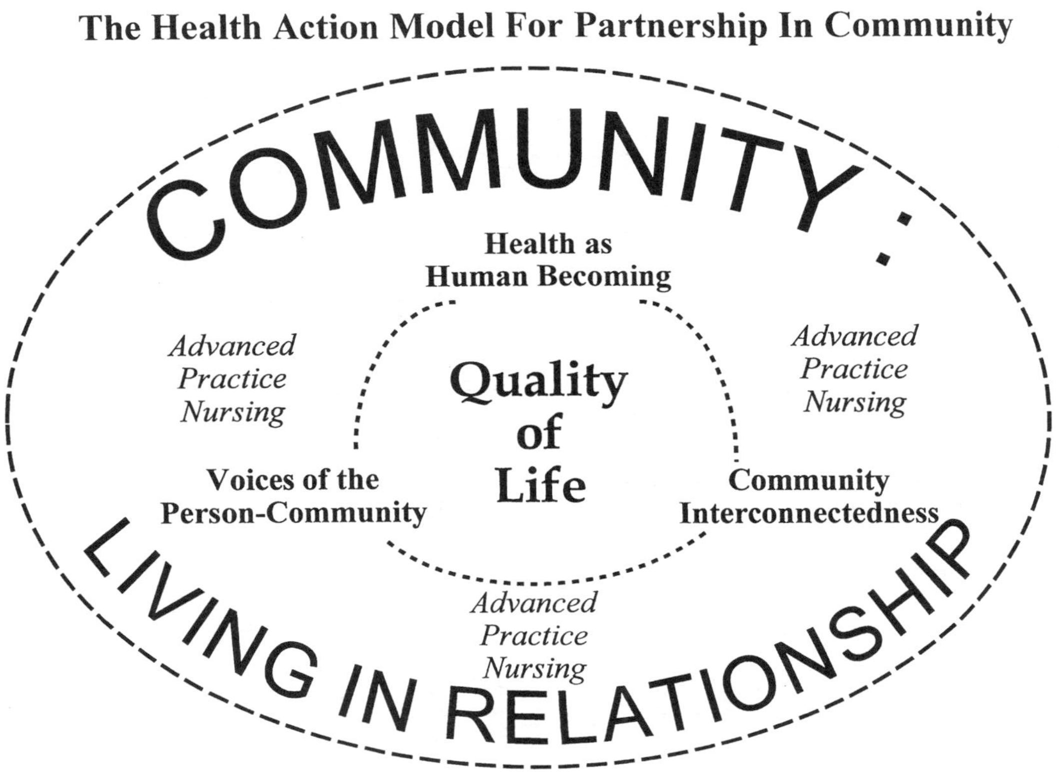

The Health Action Model For Partnership In Community

Figure 6.1. The Health Action Model for Partnership in Community. Copyright 1997 Augustana College Dept. of Nursing, Sioux Falls, SD. Reprinted with permission. *Note:* Based on Parse's (1997b) human becoming school of thought.

centers in South Dakota, North Dakota, and Minnesota. The nurse is involved in coordinating the teaching-learning activities of the primary care providers in the nine centers along with assisting them in standardizing protocols for the care of persons living with chronic illnesses, seeking input from the persons themselves. The nurse bears witness to the concerns of community and invites community to work with her in meeting aspirations for improving quality of care and quality of life. Such an invitation engages community.

Engaging community involves inviting other agencies, programs, groups, and individuals to become a partner with the community nursing model to co-create health services. These partnerships are unconventional and innovative in addressing the betterment of humankind. Along with The Dakota Network Project, another such partnership can be seen in the health action model's *Covering Kids* initiative funded by the Dakota Community Healthcare Association through a Robert Wood Johnson grant. (The focus of the grant is to sign up uninsured children in health insurance programs and to create social system changes so such a goal is possible.) The human becoming community nurse working with the Covering Kids program is involved in educating local and state outreach workers to understand children's healthcare issues. She is truly present with persons struggling with access to healthcare as they illuminate the meaning of the lack of insurance for themselves and their families. The nurse moves with them as they work toward achieving their goal of obtaining health insurance. The nurse takes part with community coalitions, including people with no insurance, recommending changes in application forms and educational processes that would streamline the insurance application process. These activities address quality of life for uninsured children and their families. All such activities in the health action model are guided by the beliefs and values depicted in its conceptual framework.

Developing a conceptual framework entails identifying the nursing theory that will guide community nursing. "Once a nursing theory is selected, creating a graphic drawing of the conceptual framework for the model is helpful in articulating the values, beliefs and focus for nursing" (Bunkers, 2002, p. 176). Beliefs and values of human becoming guide development of projects within the model, and the human becoming practice methodology (Parse, 1998) is lived by the nurses with community. Along with the human becoming framework, community's perspective of health and quality of life guides the identification of the needed operational components of the model.

Naming operational components involves clearly developing the essentials that will bring to life the objectives of the model. The HAMPIC "consists of three simultaneous integrating components—advanced practice nursing, the steering committee, and site communities" (Bunkers et al., 1999, p. 96). The intent of advanced community nursing in the HAMPIC "is to connect in true presence with persons and communities and to understand their health experiences with connections-disconnections and their hopes for changing patterns of health" (Bunkers et al., 1999, p. 96). The steering committee, composed of a representation of community agencies and persons served by the nursing model, meets quarterly to listen to and bring forward the voices of community. "These leaders have strong beliefs that community interconnectedness occurs when everyone involved has a voice" (Bunkers et al., 1999, p. 97). Site communities are partners with the health action model. "These collaborating agencies have identified a shared interest in the health and well-being of underserved populations" (Bunkers et al., 1999, p. 98). At present, site communities include Heartland House (a residential housing program for the homeless), The Good Shepherd Center (a drop-in center for the homeless), The Banquet (a city soup kitchen), Minnehaha County Welfare, The Covering Kids Initiative (Sioux Falls being the urban site for the project), The Dakota Network Project (nine community health centers covering North Dakota, South Dakota, and Minnesota), The Center For Active Generations (programs for elders in Sioux Falls), and The Sioux River Valley Community Health Center of Sioux Falls. In all of these site communities appropriate documentation systems have been created that report the activities of the projects.

Creating a documentation system for a community nursing model "must respond to the overarching objectives of the model and be consistent with the nursing theoretical framework guiding the model" (Bunkers, 2002, p. 176). Personal health description forms, community health description forms, and various other forms for evaluation of practice and nurse-community relationships have been developed in the health action model. This is an ongoing endeavor as additional projects evolve. Teaching-learning concerning the human becoming school of thought is also ongoing as new staff are added to the projects.

Participating in teaching-learning processes requires in-depth study of the nursing theory guiding the model. "It is essential to seek the involvement of nurse scholars with expertise in the nursing theoretical perspective the model selects to guide the practice" (Bunkers, 2002, p. 177). Nurses working within the health action model make a commitment to human becoming community nursing. There is continuous study of the human becoming nursing theory. Nurses attend the Institute of Human Becoming in Pittsburgh, Pennsylvania, along with receiving mentoring from a Parse scholar. Ongoing teaching-learning endeavors as well as ongoing operation of the project require obtaining funding for the model.

Obtaining funding is "one of the most challenging aspects of creating new and innovative" community models (Bunkers, 2002, p. 177). The original funding for HAMPIC was obtained from private and public sources "including Augustana College, Sioux Valley Health System Community Fund, Sioux Falls Area Foundation, Sioux Falls School District Head Start Program, and the Sioux Empire United Way" (Bunkers, 2002, p. 177). At present, some of the funding sources have shifted and include Augustana College, Sioux River Valley Community Health Center, Minnehaha County Welfare, The Dakota Healthcare Association, and The Robert Wood Johnson Foundation. Grants totaling over $280,000 have been received to help fund the model since its inception in 1997. The sustainability of this model depends on unique and diverse funding patterns, the ability to articulate the importance of this community nursing model to quality of life, and ongoing efforts in research.

Conducting research needs "a primary place of importance" within a community nursing model (Bunkers, 2002, p. 178). In the health action model, the human becoming theory and conceptual framework of the model emphasize research focusing on the meaning of lived experiences of health. An example related to the focus of research on lived experiences is the study "The Lived Experience of Feeling Cared For: A Human Becoming Perspective" (Bunkers, in press), with women struggling with economic, social, and interpersonal resources and homelessness. The findings of this research expand the human becoming theory guiding this nursing model. The findings will shed light on how these 10 women who are struggling feel cared for. Several steering committee members of the HAMPIC assisted in recruiting potential participants for the study. There was community interest in the conduction of the research and in the research findings. Such research bears witness to the lived experiences of community constituents and will be shared through presentations and publications.

Publishing the prototype of a nursing theory–guided model "informs the members of the discipline of nursing, other healthcare disciplines and the public on what is possible; it keeps the agenda for healthcare reform and change in health policy alive" (Bunkers, 2002, p. 178). The HAMPIC was featured in the book *The Outcomes Mandate* (Cohen & De Back, 1999) as an example of a nursing model that creates innovative alliances with community. "Through HAMPIC, Augustana College's Department of Nursing is seizing the opportunity to co-create a new paradigm in community nursing practice in partnership with the Sioux Falls, SD, community" (Bunkers et al., 1999, p. 92). Josephson (2000) describes her work in the health action model in "Women of Hope— Tiospaye," about a group of Native American women and others who gather with her at The Good Shepherd Center, a drop-in center for women and families seeking a safe place. Over 100 women have participated in this group, working together to focus on quality of life issues of the members. Josephson (2000) writes, "When women reconnect with Women of Hope, they are greeted with joy and welcomed as one would a family member who has been absent and missed. As one member of the group stated, 'We are family'" (p. 302). Letcher (2000) portrays living the theory of human becoming with persons visiting the Sioux River Valley Community Health Center in Sioux Falls. In *Buying Your Life* (Letcher, 2000), the story of a Sudanese refugee's encounter with experiencing the true presence of a nurse illustrates the potential inherent in bearing witness with another. Letcher (2000) writes, "John felt his 'fate [was] early death' (personal communication, June, 1998) upon our first meeting. This year he is reaching beyond the moon to find a place for Sudanese stars to shine in America" (p. 305). Another example of a published depiction of theory-guided nursing is that of Williamson (2000), who writes about her personal experience with a nurse guided by Parse's theory of human becoming in the health action model. Williamson writes in *The Test of a Nursing Theory: A Personal View*:

> I began to wonder how this theory experienced in its many forms was equipping me to be a better friend, a better community organizer, a better steering committee member. Was my quality of life improving? What had changed? My fears seemed to be less controlling. Because of the process of being honored, I gained a confidence in my abilities. (p. 127)

Publishing these moving accounts of human becoming nursing illuminates the powerful influence of theory-guided community nursing models and gives examples of hope for the betterment of humankind.

The development of the health action model is a community venture. The health action model's evolution is guided by beliefs and values of Parse's human becoming school of thought. Now, in moving on, it is time to discuss Parse's new conceptualizations of community.

Community: A Mosaic of Human Becoming

Community consists of patterns of interconnectedness (Bunkers, 2002). These patterns of interconnectedness, like an artistic mosaic, are diverse, beautiful, and ever changing in meaning. Such patterns of interconnectedness are chosen explicitly-tacitly and are lived in coconstituting personal histories. Such histories emanate the pattern of community, a mosaic of ever-changing processes of evolving. These ever-changing community concepts and processes are described by Parse, and these further illuminate meanings, patterns, and paradoxes.

Foundational Core

The human becoming principles (structuring meaning multidimensionally, cocreating paradoxical rhythms, and cotranscending with possibles) (see chapter 3, Table 3.2) underpin Parse's human becoming community change concepts.

Important for discussion about community here are several ideas inherent in the human becoming theory: health, quality of life, multidimensionality, and cocreation. *Health* is a process of living value priorities; it is a personal commitment to a lived value system (Parse, 1990). Community lives health in choosing what is important for quality of life. Health, as patterns of becoming

(Bunkers, 2002), is defined by community, and the meaning of health depicts quality of life. *Quality of life* is "what the person *there* living the life says it is" (Parse, 1994, p. 17). Quality of life is defined by community and is not evaluated by any set of societal norms, but by community itself. Quality of life is the meaning community constituents give to multidimensional lived experiences of health. *Multidimensionality* is an open, non-linear interconnectedness with the universe involving a mutual process of cocreating unlimited possibilities (Parse, 1999). Parse (1999) posits, "Multidimensional refers to the many realms of the universe that human beings live all-at-once. These realms are the explicit-tacit knowings that are interwoven, so the human's interconnectedness is with all that is" (p. 119). Multidimensionality is timeless and involves explicit-tacit knowing, freely choosing in situation, living past-present-future experiences all-at-once, living connectedness with predecessors, contemporaries, and successors, choosing values and meanings, and engaging in rhythmical paradoxical patterns of relating. "Paradoxical patterns are rhythms with two dimensions; one is usually in the foreground and the other in the background, but they are present all-at-once" (Parse, 1998, p. 23). It is in the multidimensionality of cocreated lived experiences where community meaning emerges. Cocreation is the human-universe process of choosing meaning in situation while emerging with diverse patterns of relating; these patterns of relating distinguish person from universe (Parse, 1998). "*Cocreation* refers to the coconstitutive nature of the human-universe mutual process; this means that all that is arises with the constituents of a situation" (Parse, 1999, p. 119). Understanding these cocreated, rhythmical paradoxical patterns of relating is fundamental to living the art of nursing with community, the nurse-community process. The nurse-community process is lived with true presence. "True presence is an interpersonal art grounded in a strong knowledge base reflecting the belief that each person knows 'the way' somewhere within self" (Parse, 1990, p. 139). The intent of the nurse in living true presence with community is "to bear witness to changing health patterns" (Parse, 1997a, p. 35). True presence is lived in face-to-face discussion, silent immersion (true presence without words), and lingering presence (recalling an engagement) (Parse, 1998).

Nursing is living patterns of presence with community (Bunkers, 2002). In true presence, the nurse moves with community as the meaning of community's health is illuminated. The nurse responds to the rhythms of community as paradoxical patterns of relating, such as revealing-concealing, connecting-separating, and enabling-limiting (Parse, 1998), are manifested. The nurse explores community ways of working with health patterns as community change processes of moving-initiating, anchoring-shifting, and pondering-shaping surface with community making choices concerning moving on with valued ways of living health (Parse, 2003). Patterns of presence emerge as the nurse engages community.

The principles of human becoming specify the meaning of health, quality of life, multidimensionality, and cocreation, and provide the guide for living the art of the nurse-community process. The principles are guides for developing scenarios, creating teaching-learning processes, and developing contributions to the discipline and the profession of nursing.

Developing Scenarios

The future is lived moment to moment with what was, is, and is yet to be. A way of living with the future is to create a scenario of what one imagines could be. Scenario planning is a way of imaging and considering possible futures. Scenarios help "us to take a long view in a world of great uncertainty.... [They] are stories about the way the world might turn out tomorrow" (Schwartz, 1996, p. 3). Jaworski (1998) writes concerning leading the future:

> Leadership is about creating, day by day, a domain in which we and those around us continually deepen our understanding of reality and are able to participate in shaping the future. This, then is the deeper territory of leadership—collectively "listening" to what is wanting to emerge in the world, and then having the courage to do what is required. (p. 182)

Parse's new conceptualizations of community change (moving-initiating, anchoring-shifting, pondering-shaping) give voice to what is emerging with the world. Now, we must have courage to do what is required. Further, as Jaworski (1998) states:

> I had always thought that we used language to *describe* the world—now I was seeing that this is not the case. To the contrary, it is through language that we *create* the world, because it's nothing until we describe it. (p. 178)

Jaworski's notions concerning language are similar to what Parse (1997b) suggests when she writes, "All language evolves gradually as generative ideas dawn, shifting the meaning of words and systems of words" (p. 73). Parse (2000) goes on to state, "The language used to describe aspects of an entity both reflects and cocreates evolving meanings regarding that entity" (p. 187). The language of Parse's (2003) concepts of community change create a notion of interconnectedness inherent in cocreating possibilities. The following scenario created with Parse's language will coshape the will-be of community. Creating this scenario involves articulating a "different pathway" (Schwartz, 1996, p. 3) that might exist tomorrow. In imaging it, it is already in place. The scenario guides making decisions while considering risks and possibilities.

The Scenario: Project Possibility

The time is the upcoming. The place is a conference room located in a prestigious school of nursing in The City, USA. Seated at a round oak table are representatives of the major healthcare systems in The City, providers of healthcare, consumers of healthcare, persons who lack sufficient access to healthcare, and local, state, and national political representatives. Nursing is well represented at this gathering. In fact, I, as a doctorally-prepared nurse on the faculty of a school of nursing, along with the nurse director of public health in The City, have been asked to co-chair this community planning group. The group numbers around 22 individuals. I open the meeting by stating the purpose and the name of the proposed project:

> The purpose of our gathering today is to explore the likelihood of this group writing a grant to create a nursing model addressing the safety net issues in this city. In other words, we are to discuss the potential pooling of resources and focusing of efforts on the development of adequate access to healthcare for all persons in this city. The proposed name for this project is *Project Possibility*. As you can see, the name denotes the very essence of the project. Making it feasible for all persons in The City and the surrounding area to have access to adequate healthcare is a challenge of major magnitude. However challenging, we know it involves concern for the quality of life of community, and the project holds the potential for new and exciting possibilities.

Project Possibility and the Human Becoming Concepts of Community Change

The human becoming community change concepts of moving-initiating, anchoring-shifting, and pondering-shaping are lived as Project Possibility unfolds. "Pondering-shaping is a cocreated paradoxical rhythm of community change. It is contemplating while configuring" (Parse, 2003, p. 38). At subsequent meetings, while considering the scope of Project Possibility, the group composes the structure, functions, and interconnections that bring the project to life. Considering-composing, one process of pondering-shaping community change, involves a rhythmical pattern of weaving ideas with action in inventing the new. Dialoguing-listening, another rhythm inherent in pondering-shaping community change, is lived with careful discussion of all details of the project while attending to the voices of community, the voices of those who will be the focus of nursing's presence in the project. With dialoguing-listening and considering-composing there are potentials for arriving at new ways of addressing challenges to quality of life. For example, at the third monthly meeting of the planning group for Project Possibility, five programs are identified as making up the core of the project. These programs are given the following names denoting the purposes of the programs: the

Pathways Program, the Potentiality Program, the Gathering Place Program, the Everyday Program, and the Innovations Program.

The *Pathways Program* consists of community nurses developing an ongoing referral system between the free clinics, the community health center, and doctors' offices in The City. Persons who are underinsured or who do not have health insurance are referred to the community health center or free clinic for ongoing healthcare; a pathway for access to care for underserved persons and families is being developed. The community change concept *anchoring-shifting* with the processes of *savoring-sacrificing* and *revering-liberating* are seen as nurses and other healthcare providers start moving with new patterns of referral while struggling with giving up old ways of dealing with the underserved population. "Anchoring-shifting is a cocreated paradoxical rhythm of community change. It is the persisting-diversifying that pushes-resists as community (individual or group) invents new meanings, knowing that all that was and will be is inextricably woven in the now" (Parse, 2003, p. 36). Healthcare providers delight in the fact that there is now an acknowledged care provider for the underserved (*savoring*) even though they have to give up their accustomed referral or non-referral practices (*sacrificing*). Healthcare providers and the community nurses honor that which was working in the old system (*revering*) while being free to continue to develop new ways of being with community (*liberating*).

The *Potentiality Program* is created to serve as a mentoring program and an educational program for immigrants and refugees relocating in The City. The mentors are fellow immigrants and refugees who help newly arrived persons get to know and understand The City and they refer them to agencies for necessary assistance. Mentors are assigned to persons and families for as long as the new person/family needs guidance with connecting to resources. Another aspect of the program is to facilitate the immigrant/refugee's gaining access to further education in the United States. Volunteer teachers and other professionals work with that portion of the program. The hope for this program is that with guidance and mentoring persons can reach their full potential as residents of the United States. The human becoming community concept of *moving-initiating* is forefront in creating these changes. "Moving-initiating is a cocreated paradoxical rhythm of community change. It is discarding and creating all-at-once, incarnating the value priorities of community, whether community is an individual or group" (Parse, 2003, p. 23). Moving-initiating community change has the following nine processes: tunneling, driving, laddering, boating, swimming, submarining, ballooning, motorflying, and swinging (Parse, 2003, p. 24). These processes occur all-at-once in moving-initiating community change, although some are foreground and others background with certain situations. In this situation with the *Potentiality Program*, the process of *tunneling* occurs as the planning group digs under the surface of the issues to identify the concerns of the immigrant and refugee population. The group pierces the depths in earthing and unearthing ideas for new programming to address the refugees' hopes and dreams. For example, the planning group might unearth several of the concerns of the Sudanese community. Young male refugees coming from the Sudan (referred to as *The Lost Boys*) want to become educated in America. What has been covered up or earthed until this time was the difficulty obtaining any documentation of prior education from the refugee camps. Also, differences in life experiences pose certain challenges in fitting into the U.S. educational system. Thus, *laddering*, multidimensional climbing, is necessary to address the Lost Boys' educational concerns. The planning group creates a task force that climbs up to seek the support of the superintendent of schools to find ways to facilitate schooling for all immigrants and refugees seeking further learning opportunities. The task force is recommending ways of circumventing the lack of documentation of previous education. *Laddering* multidirectionally with those with influence in the educational system and then coming back to the planning committee grounded with facts contributes to the success of the *Potentiality Program*.

Three community nursing programs are instituted to provide outreach services in The City. The *Everyday Program* is initiated to work with the three transitional housing programs in The City. The program provides a community nurse's presence at each transitional housing location one day a week. The nurse focuses on what the families see as important in the day-to-day living of health for themselves and their children. Programming to this date consists of health education on such topics as head lice and childhood fevers, health screening for children's sight and hearing, dealing with depression, and several onsite referrals to healthcare providers to address chronic health conditions of both children and parents. Personnel at the transitional housing sites state that emergency room usage by the families has decreased dramatically with the day-to-day presence of the nurse at the facilities. Similarly, the *Gathering Place Program* is initiated to work with the local soup kitchen, a drop-in center for the homeless, and the two homeless shelters in The City. Again, as in the *Everyday Program*, a community nurse spends one day a week in each of these locations focusing on what is important to persons experiencing homelessness. The nurse is present when persons gather for meals and for shelter and comfort. Likewise, the *Innovations Program* is created to work with elders in the community in creating new health programming for elders. A nurse travels between the Elder Recreation Center and three retirement villages. Elders engage with the nurse in planning projects and activities they see as important to their health and quality of life. In all three community nursing outreach programs the moving-initiating change processes of *ballooning*, *swimming*, and *driving* are lived. Ballooning involves vigilant observing of the pattern of community. An example of ballooning is when several mothers in the housing units express to the nurse serious concerns about whom to contact when their babies and small children are ill. Before this time, since they do not have health insurance, they often waited to seek care until it was necessary to take the child to the emergency room. They want the nurse to help them learn to recognize when a healthcare provider should be contacted. The nurse, working with the families and local doctors, develops a telephone call system so parents can call and describe their child's situation and symptoms and receive immediate access to a primary care provider. This telephone call system has been established at all three housing locations. Ballooning with vigilant drifting with the pattern of the whole (hearing the concern for access to care for children) "in a buoyant surgence-release" (Parse, 2003, p. 32) (creating the telephone call team) is seen in this example.

"*Swimming* is gliding with diverse currents in keeping afloat with the sureness-unsureness of moving-initiating community change" (Parse, 2003, p. 30). An example of swimming is when women in the homeless shelter come to talk with the nurse. The nurse lets the flowing current of the dialogue determine what is important to the women. There are times when the nurse treads water as a woman decides whether or not she wants to stay involved in the dialogue. Swimming with the person's rhythm cocreates an ebb and flow of ongoing discussion. This ongoing discussion often shifts to the person planning for creative health pattern change.

For the nurse working with the *Innovations Program*, what surfaces as crucial health issues for many elders is the monitoring of their blood pressure, regulating and living with diabetes, and developing plans for staying as independent as possible. The community process of driving comes into play when elders decide they want located at the Elder Center the latest *physcotronic* tracking device that monitors blood pressure, blood sugar level, and several cardiac enzymes that indicate cardiac health status. After a very simple procedure of hooking a person up to the device, a printout is produced, which the person can take and discuss with the community nurse. "*Driving* is forging directly with intensity in cocreating the shifting patterns of diversity in moving-initiating community change" (Parse, 2003, p. 27). Elders, after discussing this innovative idea with the nurse, forge ahead and solicit funds from several healthcare sources to buy this expensive device. They rapidly organize a silent auction fund-raising event at the center and, after a month of such activities, have enough money to purchase the machine. Elders' feelings of being more independent and responsible for their own health surface in the acceleration-deceleration-lateral movement of focusing on getting this new device for the Elder Center. Diverse health patterns continuously arise as the nurses work with families in the transitional housing units, with persons at the soup kitchen and shelters, and with the elder community.

All five of the community nursing programs that are part of Project Possibility have as their guide the human becoming community change concepts and processes. The human becoming beliefs concerning health, quality of life, multidimensionality, and cocreation are lived in the art of the human becoming nurse-community process. Nurses, managers of the programs, and the central planning committee engage in ongoing processes of learning about the human becoming school of thought. The community processes of *moving-initiating change*, particularly *boating, submarining, motorflying,* and *swinging,* are noted in the continuous study of human becoming theory. Boating as steering is seen as nurses and managers gain insights for keeping the programs on course in the calm-turbulence of shifting community issues. An example is when studying the nurse-community process nurses realize that being truly present with community involves honoring community as expert. Thus, nurses are present without an agenda, with the intent of bearing witness as community changes health patterns. Nurses wait to hear what is important to community. The programs are navigated with the input of community constituents.

Submarining as immersing occurs as program personnel study in great depth all aspects of the human becoming theory. An example of submarining is when five nurses from Project Possibility attend the Institute of Human Becoming in Pittsburgh to study with nurse theorist Dr. Rosemarie Rizzo Parse. They spend 2 weeks immersing in a high pressure situation uncovering what is known and not yet known about human becoming. This submarining to great depths with the theory is ongoing learning about community from a human becoming perspective.

Motorflying, as propelling persistently, occurs as project personnel continue to develop programming based on human becoming values and beliefs. For example, the nurse working in the *Gathering Place Program* is told the homeless shelters will be shut down by the mayor due to lack of funding. Her study and understanding of cocreating possibilities prompts her to explore new resources for funding the shelters. The gravity of the struggles of the homeless requires a way of weaving new funding sources with the city's. With persistence, the nurse and other Project Possibility personnel request funds from the state to add to the city's resources. Motorflying is a crucial community process in cocreating this paramount change in support for the shelter system in The City.

Swinging as soaring is experienced by personnel studying the art of human becoming. As managers, other personnel, and planning committee have come to understand the community change concepts and values of the human becoming school of thought, their presence with others is open, honoring, and inviting, and they boldly leap beyond with new ways of being with community. Many of the programs in Project Possibility are soaring to new heights as ideas for action are swingshifting with community creativity. An example is that the *Pathways Program* manager is asked to keynote an international conference on creating new community nursing models, entitled The Futuring of Community Care. Presenting the art of human becoming community nursing, as manifested in Project Possibility, is an opportunity for shifting future international potentialities.

Parse's (2003) identified themes from over 30 research studies on lived experiences, which further enlighten the human becoming concepts of community, are manifest in the ongoing work of the core planning group of Project Possibility. These themes are "(a) persistent struggling is persevering with urgent intensity; (b) anguishing solemnity is a quiet-disquiet abiding with the reverent; (c) anticipating possibles is visioning the not-yet; and (d) uplifting calmness is a buoyant serenity" (Parse, 2003, p. 97). As the core planning group continues to reflect on its purpose of providing healthcare access to community, there is present a sense of persistent struggling in persevering with an urgent intensity. We begin to explore the facts of lack of healthcare for many in the area. The group digs into the data to find out more about what is not being done for the underserved in The City. Many hours are spent trying to discern what has been and what should be. In this persistent struggle to understand there is urgency for moving with new programming. In many discussions I note an anguishing solemnity as a quiet-disquiet abiding with the reverent surfaces in the group. The group identifies, with extreme discomfort, noted inadequacies in the present care delivery systems and recognizes hurtful labeling attitudes that often keep those needing assistance with healthcare at a distance from care providers. At the same time, strengths of care delivery programs are highlighted so as to honor what has been working. Anticipating possibles in visioning the not-yet is occurring as the group moves on in planning who should be involved in writing certain grants, which agencies should be lead agencies in the expansion of Project Possibility, and what are the best ways to cocreate interagency cooperation. The creative process of visioning what can be surfaces excitement in the group. An uplifting calmness as buoyant serenity emerges as the planning group becomes confident that Project Possibility is the future of healthcare for The City, while recognizing the burdens of interagency and interdisciplinary cooperation. There is a growing understanding of each other's concerns related to healthcare. Now, at core planning sessions, laughter fills the conference room as the planning group brainstorms ways of navigating turf issues and works to develop further the community nursing model. Community change, as experienced with Project Possibility, is consistent with the themes "persistent struggling is persevering with urgent intensity," "anguishing solemnity is a quiet-disquiet abiding with the reverent," "anticipating possibles is visioning the not-yet," and "uplifting calmness is a buoyant serenity" (Parse, 2003, p. 97). Project Possibility so changes the face of healthcare locally, nationally, and internationally that new teaching-learning processes for health professionals are needed to provide new understandings of community.

Developing Teaching-Learning Processes

Teaching-learning is an ongoing process of "engaging with others in coming to know" (Bunkers, 1999, p. 227). Teaching-learning involves inviting dialogue and critique while exploring what is familiar-unfamiliar. Parse's concepts of community change give rise to new images of the familiar-unfamiliar and create new realities concerning community. Parse's (2003) definition of community along with the human becoming community change concepts and processes can serve as guides for teaching-learning (see chapter 4, Tables 4.1, 4.2, and 4.3). Displayed in Table 6.2 are examples of reflections on nurse-

---

Table 6.2. ACTIVITIES PROMOTING REFLECTIONS WITH HUMAN BECOMING
COMMUNITY CONCEPTS

The Oneness of Human-Universe Connectedness	Describe the interconnections of community. You may want to draw a picture of the community; include important environmental features, who works with whom, who communicates frequently, which persons identify themselves as leaders on certain issues and which identify themselves as followers. Including art work of the community will be important in describing its interconnectedness with the universe.
The Unique Beliefs and Values of Community	Describe beliefs and values coshaping this community, such as art, literature, and work patterns.
Personal Histories	Include community stories important in understanding health patterns. These stories can be quotations or other forms of written documents.

Human Becoming Community Change Concepts:

Moving-Initiating Community Change	Address a health pattern on which community is working with moving-initiating change. Give examples of several of the nine processes.
Anchoring-Shifting Community Change	Describe a health pattern of change that community is engaging with, in anchoring-shifting change. Give examples of the two processes.
Pondering-Shaping Community Change	Relate a dream or hope for the future that community has in pondering-shaping change. Give an example of the two processes.

The Nurse-Community Process:

	Describe and evaluate your living the art of human becoming with community.

community situations. These are a springboard for teaching-learning discussions focusing on community and nursing theory.

It is in imagining what can be that we cocreate what is. Teaching-learning from the human becoming perspective of community offers hope for new ways to address quality of life.

Continuing Development for Quality Care

Important to community nursing is the establishment of tenets for nursing, reflecting the values and the ethics of the discipline. Drawing from the human becoming school of thought (Parse, 1998), the ANA (1999) document *The Scope and Standards of Public Health Nursing Practice*, the Nursing Standards (which are consistent with the human becoming theory) developed by Sunnybrook Health Science Centre Nursing Council (1997), and from professional experience in community nursing, including developing and directing the HAMPIC (a community nursing practice model based on Parse's theory of human becoming), I composed tenets for the art of human becoming nursing with community. These human becoming tenets and indicators are concordant with the human becoming community change concepts and processes and are grounded in the ethics of the human becoming school of thought (see Table 6.3). These tenets offer a foundation for the continuous development of the art of human becoming nursing with community.

Summary

Community is an emerging mosaic of human becoming. In creating scenarios of human becoming community nursing, in developing teaching-learning processes related to community, and in directing the continuing development of quality care, one lives Parse's community change concepts of moving-initiating, anchoring-shifting, and pondering-shaping. These community change concepts with their processes immerse us with the question of "why not?" when visioning anew. With this immersion, what we imagine can be.

The vastness of the galaxy
Serene valley, mountain, turbulent sea
Nameless stranger, friend, family
I—am community.

Table 6.3. HUMAN BECOMING WITH COMMUNITY: TENETS AND INDICATORS

Tenets for Living the Art of Human Becoming Nursing With Community	Indicators of Living the Art of Human Becoming Nursing With Community
Quality of Care: The nurse engages community in describing health and quality of life.	• Community conveys that community values, beliefs, hopes, and concerns are being heard and respected. • The nurse conveys that community descriptions of health and quality of life guide the nurse-community process.
Quality of Life: The nurse focuses her/his own nursing on quality of life as defined by community.	• Community conveys that the nurse asks about quality of life. • Community conveys that the nurse asks about the goals of community.
Quality of Nursing: The nurse lives the human becoming practice methodology with community.	• Community conveys feeling respected, listened to, and actively involved in changing health patterns. • The nurse bears witness to changing patterns of community.
Quality of Performance: The nurse evaluates personal ways of living the art of human becoming and reflects on other significant professional standards and relevant statutes and regulations.	• Community conveys satisfaction with nursing. • The nurse is involved in a peer review process with other professionals.
Quality of Education: The nurse acquires and maintains current knowledge of the human becoming school of thought and other arts and sciences.	• The nurse receives formal education in human becoming (master's or doctoral education, attendance at the Institute of Human Becoming, attendance at human becoming theory conferences, ongoing study with Parse scholars). • The nurse studies the arts and other sciences.
Quality of Collegial Patterns of Relating: The nurse contributes to knowledge enhancement of peers, colleagues, and others.	• The nurse engages with peers, colleagues, and others regarding nurse-community processes. • The nurse engages in scholarly dialogue with peers, colleagues, and others.

Table 6.3 (continued)

Quality of Social Policy: The nurse engages community in anchoring-shifting patterns in cocreating social policy for health and quality of life from the community's perspective.	• Community advances and fosters social policy regarding health and quality of life. • Community conveys satisfaction with changes in social policy.
Quality of Collaborative Patterns of Relating: The nurse collaborates with community, health, and human service professionals and organizations in addressing health and quality of life issues. The nurse engages community in using all available and desired resources for health and quality of life.	• Community conveys that health and quality of life issues from the perspective of community are addressed. • Community conveys satisfaction with available resources, fostering health and quality of life from the perspective of community. • Community conveys satisfaction with the nursing presence.
Quality of Research: The nurse uses nursing theory–guided research findings and/or conducts human becoming nursing theory–guided research with community in pondering-shaping new possibles. Research findings from other disciplines inform the nurse.	• The nurse conveys that human becoming nursing theory–guided research expands nursing knowledge that guides the nurse-community process. • Professional peers convey that research findings from other disciplines inform community. • Professional peers convey that human becoming nursing research is conducted by doctorally-prepared nurse researchers.
Quality of Contributions to the Discipline and the Profession: The nurse contributes through publishing and/or presenting new knowledge concerning human becoming community nursing. The nurse fosters the human becoming perspective in organizations. The nurse participates in moving-initiating change in the discipline and the profession.	• The nurse presents ideas and human becoming models for community nursing. • The nurse publishes concerning human becoming nursing. • The nurse guides other professionals in human becoming community nursing. • The nurse engages in professional activities advancing the art and science of nursing.

References

American Nurses Association. (1999). *The scope and standards of public health nursing practice*. Washington, DC: American Nurses Publishing.

Bunkers, S. S. (1999). The teaching-learning process and the theory of human becoming. *Nursing Science Quarterly, 12*, 227–232.

Bunkers, S. S. (2002). Person and community: Coauthors of health and care. In T. Cesta (Ed.), *Survival strategies for nurses in managed care* (pp. 168–179). St. Louis: Mosby.

Bunkers, S. S. (in press). The lived experience of feeling cared for: A human becoming perspective. *Nursing Science Quarterly*.

Bunkers, S. S., Michaels, C., & Ethridge, P. (1997). Advanced practice nursing in community: Nursing's opportunity. *Advanced Practice Nursing Quarterly, 2*(4), 79–84.

Bunkers, S. S., Nelson, M., Leuning, C., Crane, J., & Josephson, D. (1999). The health action model: Academia's partnership with the community. In E. Cohen & V. De Back (Eds.), *The outcomes mandate: Case management in health care today* (pp. 92–100). St. Louis: Mosby.

Cohen, E., & De Back, V. (Eds.). (1999). *The outcomes mandate: Case management in health care today*. St. Louis: Mosby.

Davis, R. (2000). Holographic community: Reconceptualizing the meaning of community in an era of health care reform. *Nursing Outlook, 48*, 294–301.

Jaworski, J. (1998). *Synchronicity: The inner path of leadership*. San Francisco: Berrett-Koehler Publishers.

Josephson, D. (2000). Women of hope—Tiospaye. *Nursing Science Quarterly, 13*, 300–302.

Letcher, D. (2000). Buying your life. *Nursing Science Quarterly, 13*, 303–305.

Parse, R. R. (1981). *Man-living-health: A theory of nursing*. New York: Wiley.

Parse, R. R. (1987). *Nursing science: Major paradigms, theories, and critiques*. Philadelphia: Saunders.

Parse, R. R. (1990). Health: A personal commitment. *Nursing Science Quarterly, 3*, 136–140.

Parse, R. R. (1994). Quality of life: Sciencing and living the art of human becoming. *Nursing Science Quarterly, 7*, 16–21.

Parse, R. R. (1997a). The human becoming theory: The was, is, and will be. *Nursing Science Quarterly, 9*, 32–38.

Parse, R. R. (1997b). The language of nursing knowledge: Saying what we mean. In J. Fawcett & I. M. King (Eds.), *The language of nursing theory and metatheory* (pp. 73–77). Indianapolis, IN: Sigma Theta Tau.

Parse, R. R. (1998). *The human becoming school of thought*. Thousand Oaks, CA: Sage.

Parse, R. R. (1999). Community: An alternative view. *Nursing Science Quarterly, 12*, 119–121.

Parse, R. R. (2000). Language: Words reflect and cocreate meaning. *Nursing Science Quarterly, 13*, 187.

Parse, R. R. (2003). *Community: A human becoming perspective.* Sudbury, MA: Jones and Bartlett.

Rafael, A. (2000). Watson's philosophy, science, and theory of human caring as a conceptual framework for guiding community health nursing practice. *Advances in Nursing Science, 23*(2), 34–45.

Raphael, D., Steinmetz, B., Renwick, R., Rootman, I., Brown, I., Sehdev, H., Phillips, S., & Smith, T. (1999). The community quality of life project: A health promotion approach to understanding communities. *Health Promotion International, 14*(3), 197–209.

Schwartz, P. (1996). *The art of the long view.* New York: Doubleday.

Sunnybrook Health Science Centre Nursing Council. (1997). *Patient focused care standards of nursing practice.* Toronto, Canada: Author.

Williamson, G. J. (2000). The test of a nursing theory: A personal view. *Nursing Science Quarterly, 13,* 124–128.

CHAPTER 7

A SYNTHESIS OF THEMES FROM HUMAN BECOMING RESEARCH WITH THE COMMUNITY CHANGE CONCEPTS

ROSEMARIE RIZZO PARSE

Basic research discoveries arising from studies using the Parse research method (Parse, 1987, 1998, 2001b) and the human becoming hermeneutic method (Cody, 1995b, 2001; Parse, 1998, 2001b) offer understandings about humanly lived experiences. Since, from a human becoming perspective, all human experiences are community experiences, understanding of the research findings from these studies is expanded with an interpretation through the human becoming community change concepts. The human becoming view of community is that it is a oneness of human-universe connectedness incarnating beliefs and values. A contemplative reflection on the research findings from some 30 or more Parse studies uncovered four major themes that can be synthesized with the human becoming community change concepts: (a) persistent struggling is persevering with urgent intensity; (b) anguishing solemnity is a quiet-disquiet abiding with the reverent; (c) anticipating possibles is visioning the not-yet; and (d) uplifting calmness is a buoyant serenity.

Persistent Struggling Is Persevering With Urgent Intensity

Findings from research studies on lived experiences concerning the theme *persistent struggling is persevering with urgent intensity* include struggling with going along when you do not believe (Kelley, 1991), persisting while wanting to change (Pilkington, 2000), persevering through a difficult time (Allchin-Petardi, 1998), struggling with making a decision in a critical life situation (Beauchamp,1990), struggling through a difficult time (Smith, 1990), and having courage (Bournes, 2002). Participants in these studies spoke of wrestling with ideas to accommodate the thinking of others, and fighting with others while living the discomfort arising with barriers and restrictions. They immersed themselves and dug in, creating different ways of moving with a sense of security and hope, even though the unexpected loomed. Participants also spoke of pressing onward, listening to their desires, taking control, honoring and staying with their priorities, and assuming responsibility for decisions, as they drove to accomplish what was desired. They reported propelling persistently onward with others, ideas, objects, and events in moving with fear, ridicule, and stumbling blocks, as they persevered during times of embarrassment and utter frustration. The experiences described by participants in these studies were lived as community, and an understanding of them is further expanded with an interpretation through the human becoming community change concepts.

All three human becoming community change concepts (moving-initiating, anchoring-shifting, pondering-shaping) can be connected with the theme *persistent struggling is persevering with urgent intensity*. An interpretation of this theme with the *tunneling, driving, submarining,* and *motorflying* processes of moving-initiating community change expands understanding of humanly lived experiences. The urgent intensity is piercing the depths in deliberate earthing and unearthing ideas in *tunneling*. This happens as community stays with an idea and digs to find out more and more about an issue. Persevering is digging deep and staying with something. The urgent intensity of persevering is like the forging directly in *driving*. The idea of intensity is apparent in the strategies of community (individual or group) when living the value of moving with alacrity to accomplish something that is cherished. The deep immersion under pressure of *submarining* in community is like the pressure of persisting and struggling with something, knowing that the unexpected may arise. The propelling persistently of *motorflying* with community is reflective of the urgent intensity of living forceful strategies to achieve something of value.

An interpretation of the theme *persistent struggling is persevering with urgent intensity* with the *revering-liberating* process of anchoring-shifting community change expands understanding of humanly lived experiences. Persistently struggling with something intensely is a way of honoring it as something worth staying with and freeing all-at-once, a value priority arising with community. The urgent intensity is a human experience that implies honoring and freeing the valued. An interpretation of this theme with the *dialoguing-listening* process of pondering-shaping community change also expands understanding of humanly lived experiences. Dialoguing-listening is unconditional witnessing, a special way of coming to know that requires persistent struggling to understand. It is an attentiveness that requires a commitment to *be with* unfolding change in speech, silence, movement, and stillness. Community change is a persistent struggling with intensity to dialogue, listen, honor, and stay with something in digging under, forging directly, immersing deeply, and propelling persistently.

Anguishing Solemnity Is a Quiet-Disquiet Abiding With the Reverent

Findings from research studies on lived experiences concerning the theme *anguishing solemnity is a quiet-disquiet abiding with the reverent* include feeling uncomfortable (Baumann, 1996), grieving (Cody, 1995a), grieving a personal loss (Cody, 1991), grieving the loss of an important other (Pilkington, 1993), suffering (Daly, 1995), waiting (Bournes & Mitchell, 2002), and feeling alone while with others (Gouty, 1996). Participants in these studies spoke of an emptiness that was nearly unbearable when facing the loss of someone or something or when not being acknowledged, yet always with a sense of gaining an unburdening freedom. They glided in struggling with the calm-turbulent currents of uncomfortable feelings, trying to keep afloat with the sureness-unsureness of what was about to be, as they abided reverently in deeply mourning their losses. The participants spoke of cautiously shifting their plans, while honoring the remembered and flowing with the sounds, silences, movements, and stillnesses of their anguish with a sense of urgency about potentially losing track of the day-to-day in their exhaustion. The experiences described by participants in these studies were lived as community, and an understanding of them is further expanded with an interpretation through the human becoming community change concepts.

All three human becoming community change concepts (moving-initiating, anchoring-shifting, pondering-shaping) can be connected with the theme *anguishing solemnity is a quiet-disquiet abiding with the reverent*. An interpretation of this theme with the *swimming* and *ballooning* processes of moving-initiating community change expands understanding of humanly lived experiences. With swimming there is the gliding with diverse currents, like the quiet-disquiet of anguishing solemnity. This happens as community (individual or group) with diverse value priorities strives to keep afloat with the sureness and unsureness that is cocreated in abiding with the reverent. Abiding with the reverent is connected with the drifting vigilantly of ballooning. In abiding with the reverent there is an enabling-limiting communion with the pattern of the whole, and the quiet-disquiet arises with the buoyancy of the surgence-release in the shifting winds of community change.

An interpretation of the theme *anguishing solemnity is a quiet-disquiet of abiding with the reverent* with the *revering-liberating* process of anchoring-shifting community change expands understanding of humanly lived experiences. Abiding with the reverent is like honoring something of value over time, which happens as community (individual or group) weaves remembered connections and separations with new meaning moments revealed-concealed in anchoring-shifting change.

An interpretation of this theme with the *dialoguing-listening* process of pondering-shaping community change also expands understanding of humanly lived experiences. Abiding with the reverent is a way of coming to understand through cocreating the rhythms of unconditional witnessing with the sounds, silences, movements, and stillnesses alive in grieving and suffering, as these anguishing experiences permeate and surface new meanings with the pondering-shaping of community change. Community change involves an anguishing solemnity with the quiet-disquiet of abiding with the reverent, as honoring something of value comes with dialoguing-listening to understand the remembered as it is appearing now. It surfaces while gliding with the diverse currents of drifting vigilantly in communion with the pattern of the whole.

Anticipating Possibles Is Visioning the Not-Yet

Findings from research studies on lived experiences concerning the theme *anticipating possibles is visioning the not-yet* include restriction-freedom (Mitchell, 1995), hope (Parse, 1999b), considering tomorrow (Bunkers, 1998), making a promise (Milton, 1998), wanting to help another (Mitchell & Heidt, 1994), and lingering presence (Ortiz, 2001). Participants in these studies spoke of looking forward with expectancy and to living and doing the best with what they had, while planning to succeed in climbing to a different vantage point. They soared with choosing to forge optimistically with difficult situations, yet they often were suspended while waiting and moving with the winds of change, as they kept some things of value and gave up others to achieve a desire. Through speech and silence they moved with what they believed was possible. The experiences described by participants in these studies were lived as community, and an understanding of them is further expanded with an interpretation through the human becoming community change concepts.

All three human becoming community change concepts (moving-initiating, anchoring-shifting, pondering-shaping) can be connected with the theme *anticipating possibles is visioning the not-yet*. An interpretation of this theme with the *laddering* and *swinging* processes of moving-initiating community change expands understanding of humanly lived experiences. The multidirectional climbing of laddering provides a different vantage point and is connected with anticipating the not-yet. There is a multidirectional movement in laddering, like the ups and downs of hoping and wishing in imaging and anticipating possibles. Swinging as soaring in undulating suspension in community change also arises with anticipating possibles. With gusts of shifting winds there is swingshifting, and with anticipating possibles, there is an expansion of horizons as community (individual or group) is leaping beyond with possibles.

An interpretation of the theme *anticipating possibles is visioning the not-yet* with the *savoring-sacrificing* and *revering-liberating* processes of anchoring-shifting community change expands understanding of humanly lived experiences. Anticipating possibles with community change is *savoring* with delight the promise of what is wished for, while *sacrificing* that which is not a value priority for community at the moment. With the anticipation there is always the freedom to explore possibles with the restrictions set with the imaginings of personal realities. Revering-liberating is embedded in the experience of anticipating possibles as what is envisioned is honored and what is liberated are the possibles chosen as different value priorities by community.

An interpretation of the theme *anticipating possibles is visioning the not-yet* with the *considering-composing* and *dialoguing-listening* processes of pondering-shaping community change expands understanding of humanly lived experiences. Considering-composing is contemplating while birthing anew. The considering of what can be and all-at-once composing what is possible is cocreated in anticipating possibles. The considering-composing community change process (individual or group) is about aspirations, as the was and will-be are co-shaped differently as meanings change in the now moment. Dialoguing-listening is unconditional witnessing with speaking–being silent and moving–being still as ways of being with others, ideas, objects, and events. The dialoguing-listening community change process happens at the explicit-tacit realms all-at-once arising with speech, silence, movement, and stillness in living value priorities. Community change involves anticipating possibles in visioning the not-yet, while listening and dialoguing about values. What to savor and what to sacrifice while honoring value priorities arises in the freedom of multidirectional climbing, swinging, and leaping to expand horizons.

Uplifting Calmness Is a Buoyant Serenity

Findings from research studies on lived experiences concerning the theme *uplifting calmness is a buoyant serenity* include laughing and health (Parse, 1994), joy-sorrow (Parse, 1997), contentment (Parse, 2001a), serenity (Kruse, 1999), taking life day-by-day (Mitchell, 1990), feeling understood (Jonas-Simpson, 2001), feeling close (Blanchard, 1996), feeling unburdened (Huffman, 2001), being human (Cody, 1995b), and feeling peaceful (Hamalis, 2001). Participants in these studies spoke of feeling uplifted and relieved in the calm of a good life, even though there were sorrows with the joys along the way. They were contented and often laughed in pondering remembered burdens as they navigated the calm-turbulence of everyday life. They spoke of a sustaining strength and confidence when feeling the lightness of honoring and confirming who they were, as others attended to them in different ways. The experiences described by participants in these studies were lived as community, and an understanding of them is further expanded with an interpretation through the human becoming community change concepts.

All three human becoming community change concepts (moving-initiating, anchoring-shifting, pondering-shaping) can be connected with the theme *uplifting calmness is a buoyant serenity*. An interpretation of this theme with the *boating* process of moving-initiating community change expands understanding of humanly lived experiences. The steering while navigating, harnessing moments of buoyancy with the calm-turbulence of shifting waves, is reflective of the uplifting calmness that emerges in light of the unsettling times lived with community change. The uplifting calmness is always accompanied with turbulence or unrest as the familiar is shifted, and uncertainty arises when not conforming with tradition is a value priority of community (individual or group).

An interpretation of the theme *uplifting calmness is a buoyant serenity* with the *revering-liberating* process of anchoring-shifting community change expands understanding of humanly lived experiences. Uplifting calmness incarnates a lightness and buoyancy, a liberation that arises with both anchoring and shifting as meaning changes with new experiences. There is a sense of freedom that emerges with the enabling-limiting of honoring and confirming a certain value priority while all-at-once cocreating community change.

An interpretation of this theme with the *dialoguing-listening* process of pondering-shaping community change also expands understanding of humanly lived experiences. Dialoguing-listening is a call to attentiveness that is essential to pondering-shaping the possibles, and it arises with a buoyant serenity. Dialoguing-listening to understand is being unconditionally present with the sounds, silences, movements, and stillnesses of the contentment and peacefulness, and the joys and sorrows lived day-by-day during community change. Community change involves an uplifting serenity that arises in navigating the calm-turbulent rhythms of everydayness with dialoguing-listening and revering-liberating changing value priorities.

Summary

The four major themes arising from Parse research studies on lived experiences interpreted with the human becoming community change concepts (moving-initiating, anchoring-shifting, pondering-shaping) expand understanding of human experiences. This is an example of how to build unique knowledge about human experiences of health and quality of life consistent with the principles of human becoming (structuring meaning multidimensionally, cocreating paradoxical patterns, and cotranscending with possibles). Further illustrations of interpreting findings of Parse research method studies with the human becoming community change concepts and processes follow in chapters 8 and 9.

References

Allchin-Petardi, L. (1998). Weathering the storm: Persevering through a difficult time. *Nursing Science Quarterly, 11*, 172–177.

Baumann, S. L. (1996). Feeling uncomfortable: Children in families with no place of their own. *Nursing Science Quarterly, 9*, 152–159.

Beauchamp, C. (1990). *The lived experience of struggling with making a decision in a critical life situation.* Unpublished doctoral dissertation, University of Miami, FL.

Blanchard, D. (1996). *Intimacy as a lived experience of health.* Unpublished doctoral dissertation, Wayne State University, Detroit, MI.

Bournes, D. A. (2002). Having courage: A lived experience of human becoming. *Nursing Science Quarterly, 15*, 220–229.

Bournes, D. A., & Mitchell, G. J. (2002). Waiting: The experience of persons in a critical care waiting room. *Research in Nursing & Health, 25*, 58–67.

Bunkers, S. S. (1998). Considering tomorrow: Parse's theory-guided research. *Nursing Science Quarterly, 11*, 56–63.

Cody, W. K. (1991). Grieving a personal loss. *Nursing Science Quarterly, 4*, 61–68.

Cody, W. K. (1995a). The lived experience of grieving, for families living with AIDS. In R. R. Parse (Ed.), *Illuminations: The human becoming theory in practice and research* (pp. 197–242). New York: National League for Nursing Press.

Cody, W. K. (1995b). Of life immense in passion, pulse, and power: Dialoguing with Whitman and Parse—A hermeneutic study. In R. R. Parse (Ed.), *Illuminations: The human becoming theory in practice and research* (pp. 269–307). New York: National League for Nursing Press.

Cody, W. K. (2001). "Mendacity" as the refusal to bear witness: A human becoming hermeneutic study of a theme from Tennessee Williams' play *Cat on a hot tin roof.* In R. R. Parse, *Qualitative inquiry: The path of sciencing* (pp. 205–220). Sudbury, MA: Jones and Bartlett.

Daly, J. (1995). The lived experience of suffering. In R. R. Parse (Ed.), *Illuminations: The human becoming theory in practice and research* (pp. 243–268). New York: National League for Nursing Press.

Gouty, C. A. (1996). *Feeling alone while with others.* Unpublished doctoral dissertation, Loyola University Chicago.

Hamalis, P. (2001). *Feeling peaceful.* Unpublished doctoral dissertation, Loyola University Chicago.

Huffman, D. (2001). *Feeling unburdened: Research guided by Parse's human becoming theory.* Unpublished doctoral dissertation, Loyola University Chicago.

Jonas-Simpson, C. M. (2001). Feeling understood: A melody of human becoming. *Nursing Science Quarterly, 14,* 222–230.

Kelley, L. S. (1991). Struggling to go along when you do not believe. *Nursing Science Quarterly, 4,* 123–129.

Kruse, B. G. (1999). The lived experience of serenity: Using Parse's research method. *Nursing Science Quarterly, 12,* 143–150.

Milton, C. (1998). *Making a promise.* Unpublished doctoral dissertation, Loyola University Chicago.

Mitchell, G. J. (1990). The lived experience of taking life day-by-day in later life: Research guided by Parse's emergent method. *Nursing Science Quarterly, 3,* 29–36.

Mitchell, G. J. (1995). The lived experience of restriction-freedom in later life. In R. R. Parse (Ed.), *Illuminations: The human becoming theory in practice and research* (pp. 159–195). New York: National League for Nursing Press.

Mitchell, G. J., & Heidt, P. (1994). The lived experience of wanting to help another: Research with Parse's method. *Nursing Science Quarterly, 7,* 119–127.

Ortiz, M. R. (2001). *Lingering presence: A human becoming hermeneutic study.* Unpublished doctoral dissertation, Loyola University Chicago.

Parse, R. R. (1987). *Nursing science: Major paradigms, theories, and critiques.* Philadelphia: Saunders.

Parse, R. R. (1994). Laughing and health: A study using Parse's research method. *Nursing Science Quarterly, 7,* 55–64.

Parse, R. R. (1997). Joy-sorrow: A study using the Parse research method. *Nursing Science Quarterly, 10,* 80–87.

Parse, R. R. (1998). *The human becoming school of thought: A perspective for nurses and other health professionals.* Thousand Oaks, CA: Sage.

Parse, R. R. (1999a). Community: An alternative view. *Nursing Science Quarterly, 12,* 119–121.

Parse, R. R. (1999b). *Hope: An international human becoming perspective.* Sudbury, MA: Jones and Bartlett.

Parse, R. R. (2001a). The lived experience of contentment: A study using the Parse research method. *Nursing Science Quarterly, 14,* 330–338.

Parse, R. R. (2001b). *Qualitative inquiry: The path of sciencing.* Sudbury, MA: Jones and Bartlett.

Pilkington, F. B. (1993). The lived experience of grieving the loss of an important other. *Nursing Science Quarterly, 6,* 130–139.

Pilkington, F. B. (2000). Persisting while wanting to change: Women's lived experiences. *Health Care for Women International, 21*(6), 501–516.

Smith, M. C. (1990). Struggling through a difficult time for unemployed persons. *Nursing Science Quarterly, 3,* 18–28.

CHAPTER 8

HUMAN BECOMING RESEARCH ON HOPE: AN INTERPRETATION WITH THE COMMUNITY CHANGE CONCEPTS

ROSEMARIE RIZZO PARSE

Like the previous chapter, the author in this chapter discusses research findings with the human becoming community concepts, but here the content involves only findings from one particular study. The author is intent on expanding understanding of human experiences through the art and sciencing of human becoming. Consistent with this idea, Mitchell and Cody (2002) suggest that the findings arising from Parse research method studies are artfully stated and in themselves are artforms. They further state that truth and knowledge surface from engaging contemplatively with the findings from studies of lived experiences. In works on truth, Gadamer (1960/1998) purports that language constitutes the human endeavor to understand and arrive at truth. Parse (2000), in agreement, posits that language cocreates meaning and truth for the moment and that meanings change as experiences change. In an effort to discover the meaning of lived experiences through sciencing, Parse (1987) states that the art of making science is like the art of making art. Sondheim (1984) clarifies that making art requires order, design, composition, balance, and harmony. Inspired by Sondheim's work and Dewey's (1934) notion that art is the ever-changing knowledge about humans, Parse (1987) crafted the Parse research method to include structures that are linguistic abstractions, written with aesthetic simplicity and semantic clarity, illuminating the overall pattern of the whole of experiences as lived and described by participants.

In this chapter, the structures, the linguistic abstractions arrived at through multidimensionally *dwelling with* descriptions shared by Native Americans, and reported in a Parse research method study on the lived experience of hope by Parse and Kelley (1999), are considered language-art. Ten Native Americans from the Dakota tribe participated in a nine-country study on hope (Parse & Kelley, 1999). From the definition of community set forth in an earlier chapter of this book, each participant is community and the group of 10 participants is community. Dr. Lois Kelley, coinvestigator with the author on the Native American hope study (Parse & Kelley, 1999), subsequently invited a Native American artist to render an artistic expression of the findings of the study.

The author of this book invited Dr. Kelley to continue working with the artist, Larry "Running Turtle" Salazar of the Cherokee nation, to create drawings of participants' language-art (propositions arrived at from their descriptions of the lived experience of hope). What follows are the hope propositions, referred to here as language-art, from each Native American participant and the structure of hope, the drawings about the language-art by Larry "Running Turtle" Salazar cocreated with Dr. Kelley, and a discussion by this author, connecting the language-art and the drawings with the three human becoming community change concepts: moving-initiating, anchoring-shifting, and pondering-shaping.

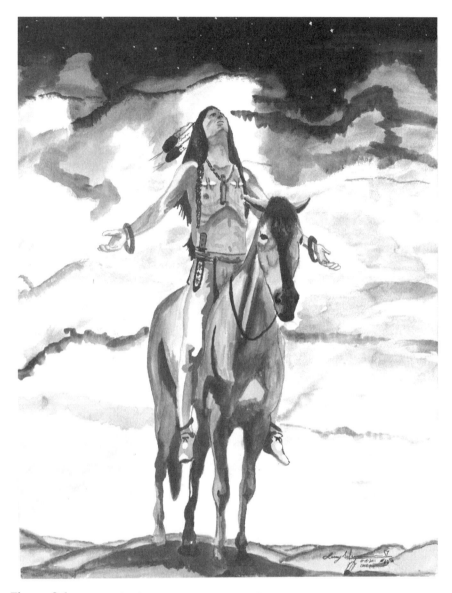

Figure 8.1. Reprinted with permission of Lois S. Kelley and Larry "Running Turtle" Salazar.

Fancy Dancer's Language-Art

> "The lived experience of hope is transfiguring with distinct sensations emerging at one with celebratory rhythms, while rising to the ethereal surfaces with relieving the commonplace amid liberating enlightenment, as contented certitude arises in meditative communion" (Parse, 1999, p. 255).

The language-art and the drawing show all three human becoming community change concepts: moving-initiating, anchoring-shifting, and pondering-shaping. With moving-initiating community change, barriers are moved with celebratory rhythms initiating a new rhythm, a giving over to the wider view of the ethereal. This is like the community process of *ballooning* where there is a vigilant drifting in viewing the pattern of the whole. The figure in the picture shows connecting-separating in moving with the rhythm, leaving the commonplace and drifting with an availability to experience the unexpected, as clouds and shifting winds loom above cocreating the ever-changing meaning of the moment.

With anchoring-shifting community change, the process of *revering-liberating* is connected with the language-art of relieving the commonplace amid liberating enlightenment. As shown in the drawing, there is an honoring and simultaneously a freeing arising with apparent new insights as the figure is living community, all he is, was, and will be. With open arms and uplifted eyes, the figure portrays the silence and stillness that appear in the language-art.

Pondering-shaping community change is connected with the drawing and language-art through the *considering-composing* community process. The idea of pushing-resisting is evident in the concerned certitude in meditative communion. The figure appears to be in intense contemplation with the hope of expected transfiguring.

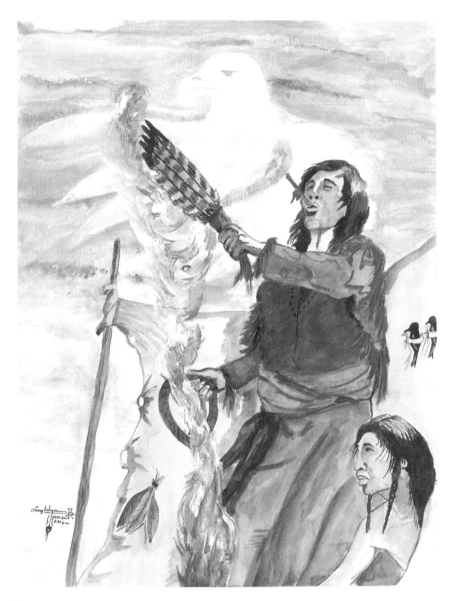

Figure 8.2. Reprinted with permission of Lois S. Kelley and Larry "Running Turtle" Salazar.

Ena's Language-Art

> "The lived experience of hope is a buoyancy in yielding with essentials despite possible futility, as commitment emerges with shifting anticipation of new possibilities, while revelation surfaces with engagements amid the tensions of encircling patterns" (Parse, 1999, p. 265).

The language-art and the drawing show all three human becoming community change concepts: moving-initiating, anchoring-shifting, and pondering-shaping. With moving-initiating community change there is the idea in the language-art of enabling-limiting in yielding with the essentials and possibles all-at-once, moving some constraints while creating others, despite possible futility. Three of the processes of moving-initiating community change (driving, laddering, and submarining) can be connected with the language-art and the drawing. The central figure (community) in the drawing appears to be whistling in a buoyant forging onward, as with the community process of *driving*. His eyes are closed as though deeply engaged in an all-enveloping imaging of new possibilities, in structuring meaning with what is known and not yet known explicitly. The deep engagement is like *submarining*, where enveloping in great depth is moving with the familiar-unfamiliar of shifting certainty-uncertainty. The reference in the language-art to encircling patterns is like the multidirectional movement of *laddering*. The encircling patterns from the language-art apparent in the drawing are the swirling clouds with eagle above, the central figure below, and small bird figures behind the central figure, portending revealing-concealing engagements with predecessors, contemporaries, and successors.

With anchoring-shifting community change, the *revering-liberating* process is connected with the language-art and the drawing through the idea of committing to envisioning new possibilities. The drawing shows the figure as connected with the encircling patterns as he is honoring the items in his hands and apparently freeing himself in transforming with a revelation.

With pondering-shaping community change, the *considering-composing* process is apparent in the language-art, and in the drawing with the central figure's closed eyes, specifying that despite possible futility, there is a ruminating and commitment to carve out different possibles, continuing the encircling patterns in moving onward. There is a deliberateness in structuring the meaning of hope while considering the certainty-uncertainty of the familiar-unfamiliar in at-once anticipating other possibles.

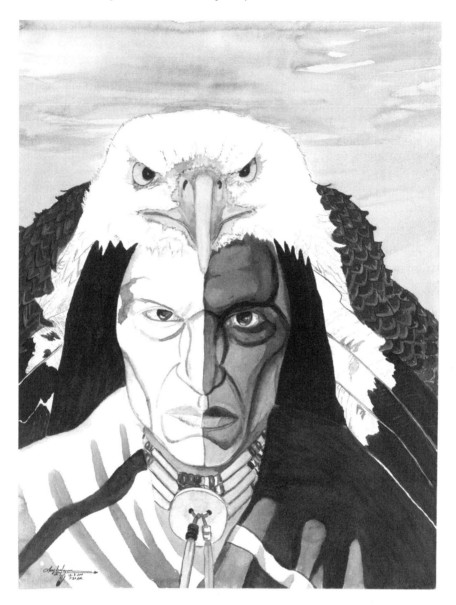

Figure 8.3. Reprinted with permission of Lois S. Kelley and Larry "Running Turtle" Salazar.

Lakota Man's Language-Art

"The lived experience of hope is astonishing, unanticipated occurrences arising amid enduring ruin, as shifting ultimate rhythms emerge with nurturing affiliations, while poignant recollections with anticipation surface in reviving legendary wisdom" (Parse, 1999, p. 266).

The language-art and the drawing show all three human becoming community change concepts: moving-initiating, anchoring-shifting, and pondering-shaping. The language-art connects with the moving-initiating community change process *swinging*. Swinging is soaring in undulating suspension awaiting unanticipated occurrences with astonishment. The figure reveals and at-once conceals the uncertainty in the dark and light sides of his face. There is a connection here with swingshifting, portending a gliding with gusts of wind, where there is always the unknown, as meanings are cocreated with moving some barriers and all-at-once initiating others. The recollecting and reviving legendary wisdom can be interpreted as the community process of *tunneling*, the earthing and unearthing of the was and will-be in the now moment. It is digging under to uncover wisdom to guide moving beyond the barrier of ruin.

With anchoring-shifting community change, the language-art shows enduring with emerging shifting rhythms as in the drawing, where dark and light sides of the figure's face show constancy yet change. The *revering-liberating* community process can be seen here as the eagle figure is hugging the central figure in a nurturing way as if revering the enduring cherished and all-at-once liberating a move with different possibles.

With pondering-shaping community change, the language-art refers to poignant recollections with anticipation, and this is shown in the somber-faced figure in the drawing. *Considering-composing* is the predominant community process shown here, as the recollections of the familiar cocreate the meaning of the unfamiliar moments arising in the unanticipated occurrences. There is a sense of certainty and uncertainty in the figure as legendary wisdom is sought as essential for hope.

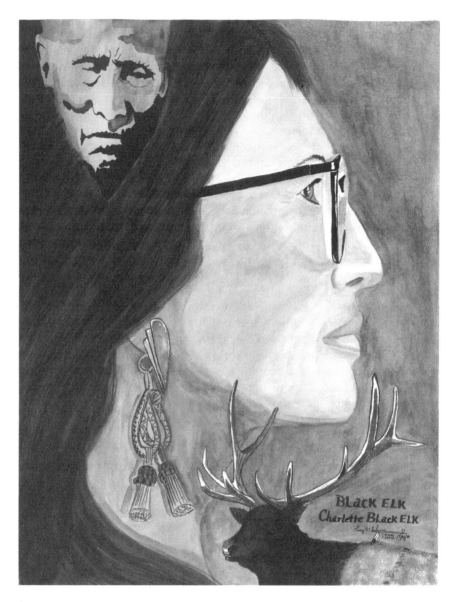

Figure 8.4. Reprinted with permission of Lois S. Kelley and Larry "Running Turtle" Salazar.

Charlotte Black Elk's Language-Art

"The lived experience of hope is transfiguring oneness arising with en-during immersion, while shifting anticipation of the was and will-be emerges amid incumbencies, as exposing treasured affiliations arises in perpetuating the venerated" (Parse, 1999, p. 263).

The language-art and drawing show all three human becoming community change concepts: moving-initiating, anchoring-shifting, and pondering-shaping. With moving-initiating community change, there is transfiguring oneness in the language-art that portrays the changing of the now with the what was and the will-be. The woman looks through glasses as if envisioning possibles, yet remembering the elder and the elk as treasured affiliations. The connection can be made to the community process of *boating*, which is steering while navigating the familiar and unfamiliar, always aware of the what was, is, and will-be in cocreating the meaning that changes when situations change.

Anchoring-shifting community change points to enduring immersion with shifting anticipation. This is evident in the language-art and in the drawing with the elder figure appearing as a symbol of anchoring the remembered for the woman. The woman looking onward can be interpreted as shifting with anticipation to persist yet change in times of difficulty. This is consistent with the *revering-liberating* community process. It is as if the woman figure reveres and honors the elder perpetuating a tradition, yet looks beyond with anticipation, a freeing vision of hope for the possibles.

With pondering-shaping community change the language-art and drawing give testimony to the woman figure as considering and at-once composing. The venerated elder appears to be in her thoughts as she contemplates the possibles. Like the *considering-composing* community process, there is an affirming of the was and will-be all-at-once in the now.

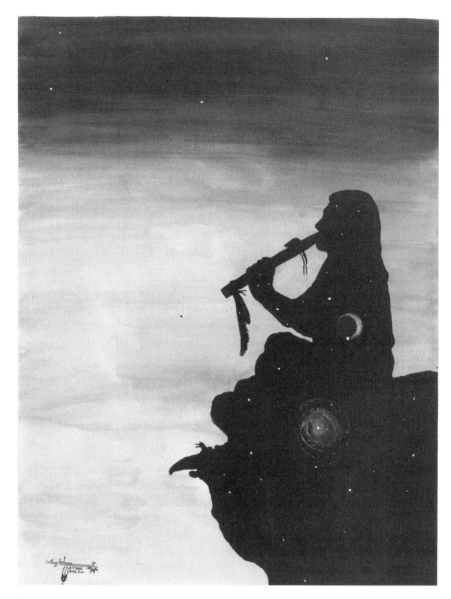

Figure 8.5. Reprinted with permission of Lois S. Kelley and Larry "Running Turtle" Salazar.

Wacantekiye Win's Language-Art

> "The lived experience of hope is a spirited fruition emerging with shift-
> ing arduous positionings, as essential mutuality arises with the yield-
> ing of acrimony, while elevating preferred polestars surfaces with
> prized legendary wisdom" (Parse, 1999, p. 268).

The language-art and the drawing show all three human becoming community change concepts: moving-initiating, anchoring-shifting, and pondering-shaping. Moving-initiating community change is evident in the language-art of shifting arduous positionings, which is suggestive of removing barriers and all-at-once creating new ones. Like the community process of *ballooning*, a drifting vigilantly, the flute player cocreates a buoyant surgence-release as different meanings arise in the melody of the moment. The position of the figure at the edge of a cliff looking outward suggests imaging possibles, languaged in the music.

Anchoring-shifting community change is shown in the flute-playing figure, who appears to be grounded on the cliff, yet transforming the moment with music. In the language-art, the valuing of legendary wisdom anchors and confirms elevation of preferred polestars with remembered traditions. This is like the *savoring-sacrificing* community process where what is important is savored and what is less important is sacrificed. Here, the essential mutuality is savored with the yielding of acrimony in structuring a different reality with hope for the will-be.

Pondering-shaping community change is evident in the spirited fruition of the language-art and in the drawing. The spirited fruition is suggestive of the community processes of *considering-composing* and *dialoguing-listening*. For considering-composing there is a deliberate aliveness evoked with accomplishing something, the playing of the music. The flute player is deliberately composing different possibilities as meaning is cocreated there on the cliff in the night air. The figure is dialoguing with the music of the flute and listening to the composition, affirming what was and what will be in the now moment.

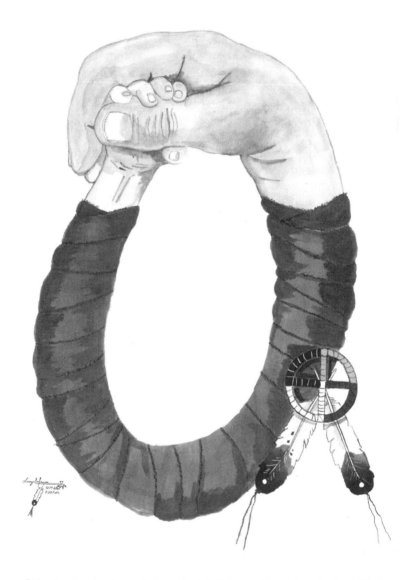

Figure 8.6.   Reprinted with permission of Lois S. Kelley and Larry "Running Turtle" Salazar.

Stone Healer's Language-Art

"The lived experience of hope is transfiguring certitude emerging with coalescing the cherished, as all-encompassing mutuality arises with the intermingling of naïveté with sagacity, while unconditional engaging with endowments surfaces with recollecting procreatory affiliations" (Parse, 1999, p. 257).

The language-art and the drawing show all three human becoming community change concepts: moving-initiating, anchoring-shifting, and pondering-shaping. With moving-initiating community change, the embracing of the small hand of the child and large hand of the elder in a circle of oneness is suggestive of a mutual transfiguring in a seamless evolving in sharing meanings as truths over generations. There is an apparent pattern of removing and initiating constraint as in the community process of *swimming*, which is defined as gliding with diverse currents in keeping afloat. The circle of holding hands is confirming what is valued and is a symbol of coalescing the cherished. There is evidence of a mutuality where elder and younger cocreate wisdom, affirming their being in the meanings of the moment.

Anchoring-shifting community change is connected to the language-art and the drawing through the intermingling of naïveté (the young hand) with sagacity (the elder hand). The anchoring in the sage brings knowledge and tradition to the shifting meaning in the naïve one. This is suggestive of *revering-liberating*, which arises in honoring and freeing. The clasped hands are not chains but, rather, a reverent unconditional engaging of endowments that cocreate the hope of freeing possibilities.

Pondering-shaping community change is evident in the language-art with recollecting procreating affiliations and in the drawing with the unbroken circle of younger with elder. There is evidence of the *considering-composing* community process as the hands are deliberately clasped with the small fingers holding onto the thumb of the larger hand as if together cocreating the remembered and possible all-at-once. The shaping of the possibles arises with the imaginings of community, individual with group, as naïveté and sagacity are one.

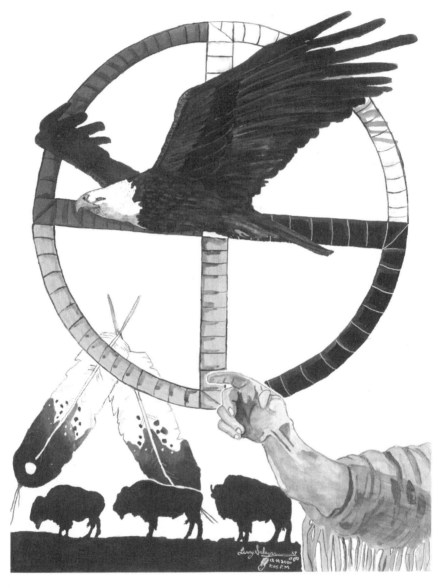

Figure 8.7. Reprinted with permission of Lois S. Kelley and Larry "Running Turtle" Salazar.

Buffalo Hunter's Language-Art

"The lived experience of hope is shifting with the new amid steadfast certitude that surfaces with a wondering quiet, as anticipation with emerging affiliations expands at one with impudent possibilities, while prevailing venerated symbols awaken the beneficent" (Parse, 1999, p. 258).

The language-art and the drawing show all three human becoming community change concepts: moving-initiating, anchoring-shifting, and pondering-shaping. Moving-initiating community change is depicted in the language-art in the idea of emerging affiliations expanding with impudent possibilities and with the figure in the drawing pointing beyond to what is not yet visible. These are suggestive of the changing of some barriers with at-once cocreating new ones. This is like the community process of *boating*, which is steering while navigating the unknown calm-turbulence of shifting waves and winds. The emerging affiliations in the language-art and the eagle floating on the wind in the drawing are suggestive of harnessing moments of buoyancy, cocreating new experiences and all-at-once new meanings.

Anchoring-shifting community change is evident in the language-art and the drawing. In the language-art, the shifting with the new amid steadfast certitude and, in the drawing, the figure pointing to an unknown while the eagle in flight oversees the buffalo on the horizon are suggestive of the community process of *savoring-sacrificing*. The steadfast truth is savored, yet there is shifting, a sacrificing to move beyond. The threads of constancy are in the prevailing symbols guarded by the buffalo, as the changing diversity with eagle in flight prefigures and awakens the hope for new possibilities.

Pondering-shaping community change is evident in the language-art and the drawing with the reference to wondering quiet in anticipation and with the figure pointing beyond and the eagle overhead. These are suggestive of the community process *considering-composing*. The wondering quiet suggests profound consideration, and the anticipation is an envisioning of possibles, shaping change in cocreating meaning with transforming the familiar-unfamiliar.

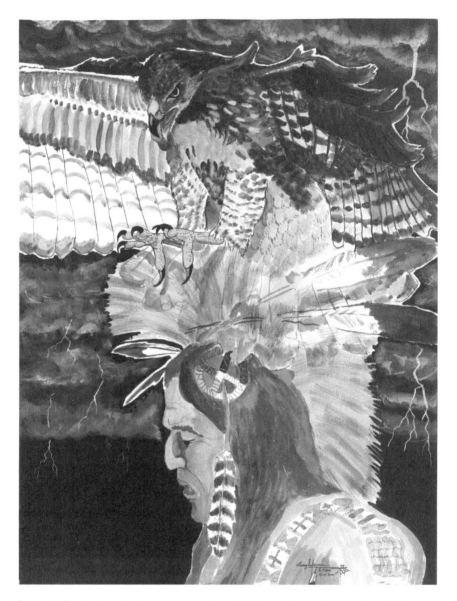

Figure 8.8. Reprinted with permission of Lois S. Kelley and Larry "Running Turtle" Salazar.

Chaske's Language-Art

"The lived experience of hope is a metaphysical shifting that arises with the vigor of ineffable reverence, while diverse meditative rhythms emerge with a chosen stance, as engaging venerated symbols surface with fortitude amid quietude" (Parse, 1999, p. 259).

The language-art and drawing show all three human becoming community change concepts: moving-initiating, anchoring-shifting, and pondering-shaping. Moving-initiating community change is evident in the language-art with the idea of metaphysical shifting, which is a way of removing and creating barriers all-at-once. In the drawing, there is a metamorphosis unfolding in the figure as the spirit of the hawk hovers above. This can be connected with the community process of *swinging*. Swinging is soaring in undulating suspension with to-and-fro swingshifting, which is like metaphysical shifting in that it refers to a bold leaping beyond the moment with hope for the new. There are undulating rhythms in swingshifting that arise with the gusts of wind cocreating the shifting experience, changing the meaning of the moment, thus reality.

Anchoring-shifting community change is shown in the reference to vigorous reverence for venerated symbols. The symbols mentioned in the language-art and shown in the drawing are the anchors with tradition, yet with the diverse rhythms, meanings of the symbols shift with new experiences. The community process of *revering-liberating* is evident as the figure, near the lightning in the sky, marks a moment of transformation in honoring with ineffable reverence what he was, is, and will be as the hawk-spirit lingers overhead.

Pondering-shaping community change is evident in the quietude and fortitude arising with the diverse meditative rhythms in the language-art and the intense concentration apparent on the face of the figure. This is consistent with the community process of *considering-composing* as the figure appears to be intensely concentrating or deliberating, while all-at-once composing a different way of becoming.

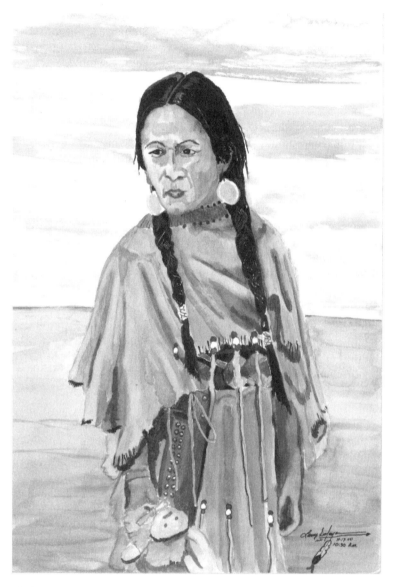

Figure 8.9. Reprinted with permission of Lois S. Kelley and Larry "Running Turtle" Salazar.

Winyan's Language-Art

"The lived experience of hope is an astonishing realization emerging with the arduous, as discerning judgments arise with the disjoining of legendary wisdom, while fortifying treasured expressions with affiliations surface with uncovering the beauteous" (Parse, 1999, p. 261).

The language-art and drawing show all three human becoming community change concepts: moving-initiating, anchoring-shifting, and pondering-shaping. With moving-initiating community change, there is in the language-art the astonishing realization with uncovering the beauteous. This is like the community process of *tunneling*; it is earthing and unearthing to make the beautiful visible. The earthing-unearthing is moving some barriers while at-once creating new ones. The figure of the woman with a doll and mature face incarnates the idea of living with the arduous in removing or disjoining the legendary wisdom through discerning judgments, cocreating changes in the meaning of tradition with living new experiences.

Anchoring-shifting community change is evident in the reference in the language-art to fortifying treasured expressions and disjoining legendary directions and in the drawing with the woman clinging to the doll, a prize of her youth. This is like the *savoring-sacrificing* community process. The figure appears to be savoring the treasured of her youth as an anchoring with tradition while at-once shifting through sacrificing legendary wisdom, cocreating hope for the not-yet.

Pondering-shaping community change is evident in the realization that arises with making discerning judgments. This is like the community process of *considering-composing*. The figure in deep contemplation shows deliberate choices in shaping new wisdom, affirming what was legendary and what is possible all-at-once.

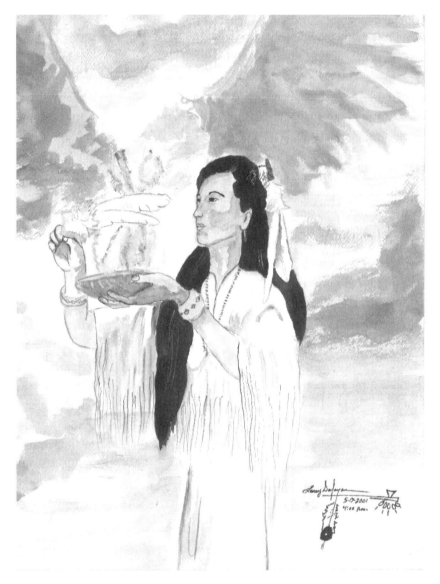

Figure 8.10. Reprinted with permission of Lois S. Kelley and Larry "Running Turtle" Salazar.

High Eagle's Language-Art

"The lived experience of hope is propelling certitude with transfiguring affirmation surfacing amid enduring adversity, while embracing the ponderous covenant arises in yielding with the cherished, as enlivened affiliations emerge with nurturing legendary wisdom" (Parse, 1999, p. 262).

The language-art and the drawing show all three human becoming community change concepts: moving-initiating, anchoring-shifting, and pondering-shaping. Moving-initiating community change is evident in the reference in the language-art to propelling certitude with transfiguring affirmations and in the drawing of the woman with an ethereal eagle figure overhead, portending removing barriers and at-once initiating new ones. The propelling certitude and apparent sacred offering by the figure are like the community process of *motorflying*, which is a persistent movement with profound intent, affirming certainty in light of the uncertainty ever present when shifting realities.

Anchoring-shifting community change is evident in the reference to nurturing of legendary wisdom while enduring adversity and in the drawing where the figure is displaying a customary ritual. There is a sense of the constant, yet a yielding with the cherished that portends a shifting with the possibles that arises with any transfiguring. It is like the community process of *revering-liberating* where the legends are honored as the cherished and the anticipated transfiguring is freeing. There is hope in shifting with adversity as a new covenant cocreates meanings that structure a different reality.

Pondering-shaping community change is evident in the reference to embracing the ponderous covenant and in the meditative appearance of the figure in the drawing. It is like the community process of *considering-composing* where there is a deep contemplation of the sacred order with an all-at-once birthing anew. The new covenant is the cherished connecting-separating in cocreating meaning with enlivened affiliations.

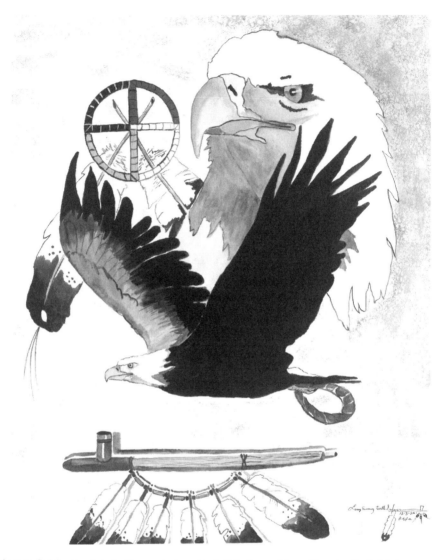

Figure 8.11. Reprinted with permission of Lois S. Kelley and Larry "Running Turtle" Salazar.

Language-Art of the Structure of Hope

"The lived experience of hope is transfiguring enlightenment arising with engaging affiliations, as encircling the legendary surfaces with fortification" (Parse, 1999, p. 256).

This is the structure of the lived experience of hope for the community of 10 Native Americans who participated in the Parse study on hope. The structure was synthesized from the 10 propositions created from their descriptions.

The language-art and the drawing for the structure of hope show all the community human becoming change concepts: moving-initiating, anchoring-shifting, and pondering-shaping. The language-art with reference to transfiguring enlightenment and fortification of the legendary, and the drawing with an eagle in flight with traditional native symbols are suggestive of ongoing community change. The new insights through the enlightenment are shifting the meaning of the legends and symbols, yet the legends are anchored in the remembered, affirming and fortifying the was, is, and will-be as all-at-once present in the ever-changing now. With transfiguring, there is a transforming that portends a moving of some barriers and all-at-once initiating others, as engaging with community affiliations (all predecessors, contemporaries, and successors) cocreates rhythmical patterns that reveal and at-once conceal value priorities, and enable and at-once limit possibilities. There is a certainty and uncertainty with the transfiguring of encircling the legendary, since the notion of conforming with tradition arises with change and awakens conflict in cotranscending with imagined possibles. The enlightening arises with pondering-shaping, a deep contemplation in connecting-separating with the imagined in structuring meanings of hope that are lived in speech, silence, movement, and stillness.

Summary

In this chapter, the author interpreted, from the perspective of the human becoming community change concepts, the language-art (propositions) from the 10 Native American participants in a nine-country Parse research method study on hope and the drawings by a Native American artist. In the interpretation with the community change concepts a light is shed on the meaning of hope as lived and described by this community. The ideas arising from moving-initiating, anchoring-shifting, and pondering-shaping bring to the fore the importance of viewing individual and group as community of oneness, a human-universe interconnectedness incarnating beliefs and values. The community change concepts with their processes are present in everyday situations as humans structure meaning, cocreate paradoxical patterns, and cotranscend with the possibles in living health and quality of life.

References

Dewey, J. (1934). *Art as experience*. New York: Perigee Books.
Gadamer, H.-G. (1998). *Truth and method* (2nd rev. ed.) (J. Weinsheimer & D. G. Marshall, Trans.). New York: Continuum. (Original work published 1960)

Mitchell, G. J., & Cody, W. K. (2002). Ambiguous opportunity: Toil for the truth of nursing art and science. *Nursing Science Quarterly, 15*, 71–79.

Parse, R. R. (1987). *Nursing science: Major paradigms, theories, and critiques.* Philadelphia: Saunders.

Parse, R. R. (1999). *Hope: An international human becoming perspective.* Sudbury, MA: Jones and Bartlett.

Parse, R. R. (2000). Language: Words reflect and cocreate meaning. *Nursing Science Quarterly, 13*, 187.

Parse, R. R., & Kelley, L. S. (1999). Hope as lived by Native Americans. In R. R. Parse, *Hope: An international human becoming perspective* (pp. 251–272). Sudbury, MA: Jones and Bartlett.

Sondheim, S. (1984). Sunday. In J. Lapine [book] & S. Sondheim [music and lyrics], *Sunday in the park with George: A musical.* New York: Dodd, Mead, & Company.

CHAPTER 9

STORIES OF COURAGE AND CONFIDENCE: AN INTERPRETATION WITH THE HUMAN BECOMING COMMUNITY CHANGE CONCEPTS

DEBRA A. BOURNES

The purpose of this chapter is to explore the meaning of the findings from two research studies (Bournes, 2002; Bournes & Parse, 2002) in light of the human becoming community change concepts: moving-initiating, anchoring-shifting, and pondering-shaping (Parse, 2003). This exploration provides new insights about the individual stories and collective findings describing the lived experiences of having courage (Bournes, 2002) and feeling confident (Bournes & Parse, 2002) that emerged from descriptions given by persons living with a spinal cord injury. It is grounded in my beliefs about the human-universe-health process, my experiences in research and practice, my search for new ways of sharing what I have learned about human experience from talking to the men and women who have participated in my research. My hope is that I can enhance understanding of nursing knowledge and provide insight about persons' stories of universal human experiences that may help nurses, and others, to be with communities (individuals or groups) in ways they say are helpful for their health and quality of life.

Parse (2003) defines community as "a oneness of human-universe connectedness incarnating beliefs and values" (p. xi). It is an "indivisible, unpredictable, and ever-changing" (Parse, 2003, p. 23) process of living in relation with others, ideas, objects, and events in this universe and beyond. Community is "coconstituted with all the personal histories of the individuals who are [have been, and will be] present" (Parse, 1999, p. 119). From Parse's definition, the participants in these studies are community. The finding of each study is the cocreated meaning of the lived experiences that emerged with the interconnectedness of the unique personal histories of all participants. Each participant is also community. The descriptions of the lived experiences that persons shared are unique incarnations of the was, is, and will-be shining forth in the moment and cocreated with predecessors, contemporaries, and successors. The individual (community) descriptions and the synthesized descriptions of both having courage and feeling confident, when interpreted in light of the human becoming community change concepts (moving-initiating, anchoring-shifting, pondering-shaping), expand knowledge about human becoming and contribute to understanding of humanly lived experiences.

Research Participant Group as Community

Feeling confident and *having courage* are both universal lived experiences that can be described by everyone, in some way, in relation to their own lives. They are particularly vivid experiences for persons who have had to make ways to live the challenging changes after a spinal cord injury. Twenty persons who were living at home after having a spinal cord injury agreed to share with the researchers their experiences, metaphors, and symbols of either having courage (Bournes, 2002) or feeling confident (Bournes & Parse, 2002). In this section, insights and themes that arose from reflectively contemplating the major findings discovered about the experiences of having courage and feeling confident are shared and further illuminated in light of Parse's (2003) human becoming community concepts. The reports of both Parse research method (Parse, 1987, 1998, 2001) studies have been documented in detail elsewhere (Bournes, 2002; Bournes & Parse, 2002). What follows is a brief summary of the findings and a detailed look at what the researchers learned about community from interpreting the findings in light of the human becoming community change concepts.

Six core concepts, three about having courage and three about feeling confident, were discovered (see Table 9.1). Core concepts are extracted and synthesized from dialogical engagements with the study participants. They are the central ideas about either the experience of having courage, or the experience of feeling confident, which were described, in some way, by every participant (Parse, 2001). The core concepts from each study were synthesized into the following structures: (a) The lived experience of having courage is a fortifying tenacity arising with triumph amid the burdensome, while guarded confidence emerges with the treasured (Bournes, 2002); and (b) Feeling confident is a buoyant assuredness amid unsureness that arises with sustaining engagements while persistently pursuing the cherished (Bournes & Parse, 2002).

Interpretation of these structures in light of the human becoming community change concepts sheds a different light on the meaning of the lived experiences and on community. The structures of having courage and feeling confident, as interpreted with the human becoming community change concepts, illuminate participants' (community's) descriptions of persistence,

Table 9.1. CORE CONCEPTS OF HAVING COURAGE AND FEELING CONFIDENT

Phenomenon	Core Concept	Meaning of Core Concept
Having Courage*	Fortifying Tenacity	Unyielding enlivening willfulness to persist.
	Triumph Amid the Burdensome	Achievement and success amid the tribulations encountered in day-to-day living.
	Guarded Confidence With the Treasured	Hesitant assuredness with expectations of cherished people, activities, hopes, and ideas.
Feeling Confident**	Buoyant Assuredness Amid Unsureness	An enriching and exhilarating feeling of surety experienced together with the unsettling tentativeness in wavering with ambiguity.
	Sustaining Engagements	Feeling good about connections with activities, accomplishments, and relationships.
	Persistently Pursuing the Cherished	A determined and ardent quest to achieve what is personally important.

*Bournes (2002)
**Bournes and Parse (2002)

sureness amid unsureness, and commitment to pursuing value priorities. The core concepts that arose in both studies capture the community's descriptions of treasured (Bournes, 2002) or cherished (Bournes & Parse, 2002) people, ideas, objects, and events, as integral with feeling confident and having courage in day-to-day living while cocreating continuous life change. The community, the participants from both studies, described either having courage or feeling confident in light of the tenacity (Bournes, 2002) and persistence (Bournes & Parse, 2002) with which they pursued what they wanted, despite the obstacles and barriers that cocreated uncertainty and made real the possibility of not achieving goals.

Moving-Initiating Community Change

The human becoming community change concept *moving-initiating* is "discarding and creating [barriers and constraints] all-at-once.... Community barriers are reality structures, the cocreated meanings of the moment that are discarded and created to conform or not conform with traditional value priorities" (Parse, 2003, pp. 23–24). The participants (community) in these studies spoke of the ways confidence and courage cocreated ardent, determined, and unyielding quests to achieve what was important despite barriers cocreated by people, ideas, objects, and circumstances. Participants talked about persistence in moving barriers, such as the ridicule of others who told them they would not or could not accomplish their goals, the fears and uncertainties connected with learning new things, and actual objects that made it difficult to navigate. Consistent with Parse's (2003) view that obstacles and barriers are not removed without creating new ones, this community spoke of both the opportunities created by removing barriers and the restrictions, or new obstacles, created by doing so.

For example, this community described having courage and feeling confident to venture away from home and shared details about, for instance, what it took to triumph over the fear of going out, returning to work, or making new friends; yet, when participants did go out, go to work, or try to meet new people, there were difficulties with encountering physical obstacles, being unable to do desired work, and being treated differently by some people who, when approached, seemed afraid to shake hands. The theme *unyielding resolve* describes the participants' (community's) descriptions of *tenacity* and *persistence* in striving for what they wanted, despite *burdensome* obstacles and barriers (see Table 9.2). *Unyielding resolve* can be further illuminated through an interpretation with four of Parse's (2003) nine processes of moving-initiating community change: swinging, tunneling, motorflying, and driving.

The new obstacles that arose with participants' (community's) *unyielding resolve* to strive for what they wanted often cocreated a *swinging* process in which they would move back and forth, at times describing having courage and feel-

Table 9.2. COMMUNITY THEMES

Ideas From Structures of the Lived Experience		Community Theme	Human Becoming Community Change Concept
Having Courage	Feeling Confident		
Tenacity, Triumph Amid the Burdensome	Persistently Pursuing	Unyielding Resolve	Moving-Initiating
Fortifying	Buoyant, Sustaining Engagements	Inspiriting Involvements	Anchoring-Shifting
Guarded Confidence	Assuredness Amid Unsureness	Certainty-Uncertainty	Pondering-Shaping

ing completely confident with carrying on with certain ventures, and at other times describing fear and uncertainty about those same ventures. This to-and-fro movement of having courage–being afraid, and feeling confident–feeling unsure emerged with the community's descriptions of having courage and feeling confident as "undulating rhythms" (Parse, 2003, p. 34) that cocreate possibilities for "leaping beyond" (Parse, 2003, p. 34) fears and doubts about what would happen, in order to create ways to live what was important.

In some instances, community shared examples of having courage or feeling confident as an *unyielding resolve* to leap beyond with cherished possibilities through *tunneling*, that is, "digging under, piercing" (Parse, 2003, p. 25) the superficial realms of patterns of relating with others, ideas, objects, and events, deliberately unearthing the words and actions of some people and ideas that were holding them back for the purpose of showing themselves and others that their doubts were wrong, yet earthing connections with other people, ideas, and circumstances that were not affirming and that made the possibility of not achieving goals explicit. Through the descriptions of having courage and feeling confident that led to the theme *unyielding resolve*, participants (community) illuminated *motorflying*, that is, what it is like to propel persistently "in grave situations where achieving something of value is at risk" (Parse, 2003, p. 33). Community shared examples of falling down and getting back up, surviving and going forward, and being willing to keep on trying, since to do otherwise would mean not accomplishing what was desired. Amid the descriptions of having courage and feeling confident that connect with the moving-initiating community change process *motorflying*, the participants (community) also described experiences of having courage and feeling confident that illustrate the process of *driving*. The community's *unyielding resolve* emerged in examples of "forging directly with [the] intensity" (Parse, 2003, p. 27) of not being able to quit once they had started taking charge, moving onward, and getting their lives in shape. Several participants (community) talked about doing this with such an intensity that, when they think about it now, they find hard to believe (Bournes & Parse, 2002). In addition, participants shared that the experience of either having courage or feeling confident to pursue value priorities (through the swinging, tunneling, motorflying, and driving processes of moving-initiating community change) was inextricably connected with invigorating and emboldening involvements with others, ideas, and projects cocreated moment-to-moment with all that was, is, and will be.

Anchoring-Shifting Community Change

The human becoming community change concept *anchoring-shifting* is "the persisting-diversifying that pushes-resists as community ... invents new meanings, knowing that all that was and will be is inextricably woven in the now" (Parse, 2003, p. 36). The participants (community) in these two studies spoke about the ways that either having courage or feeling confident to explore, pursue, and learn new ways of living was intensely connected with fortifying (Bournes, 2002) and sustaining (Bournes & Parse, 2002) immersions with what was happening in the moment; with memories of people, ideas, objects, and activities that they used to treasure; and with hopes and plans for the future. The community spoke about experiences of having courage or feeling confident as the strength and inspiration drawn from "threads of constancy" (Parse, 2003, p. 36) intertwined with the changing day-to-day realities of life. For some, the threads of constancy were the love and support of family members and friends who helped them have courage or feel confident to pursue dreams. Others shared examples of "anchoring the now with the remembered and the not-yet" (Parse, 2003, p. 36) in descriptions of feeling a rush of confidence when, for instance, looking at photographs of themselves and their families engaged in activities that they had felt confident with prior to their injury. Still others spoke of the courage and confidence to try new things that was cocreated with pride in day-to-day achievements and successes. The theme *inspiriting involvements* arises with the community's descriptions of the fortifying, buoyant, and sustaining engagements integral with having courage and feeling confident with the cherished (see Table 9.2). It can be further illuminated by, and can shed light on, the two major processes of anchoring-shifting community change: *savoring-sacrificing* and *revering-liberating*.

"*Savoring-sacrificing* is delighting in and all-at-once foregoing something of value in anchoring-shifting community change" (Parse, 2003, p. 37). Participants in these two studies described having courage and feeling confident in connection with anchoring themselves with *inspiriting involvements* with others, ideas, objects, and events. The community spoke of relishing moments when they were able to do things for themselves and for others that made them feel good and when they were able to accomplish even the smallest things independently. For some, this meant having courage or feeling confident when engaging in sports or traveling. Some talked about having courage and feeling confident in light of the pleasure and satisfaction experienced from receiving affirmation from others who listened to what they had to say, or who felt inspired by their accomplishments. There were also instances where community described having courage and feeling confident to forego *inspiriting involvements* that were "originally delighted in" (Parse, 2003, p. 37). Descriptions of sacrificing some possibilities in order to realize others included, for instance, accounts of refraining from asking family members or friends to be there all the time, or to help with certain tasks that may once have been savored, since the importance of this help shifted—waning as new experiences cocreated different possibilities for *inspiriting involvements* with those same people. All participants (community) described changing patterns of relating, with reverence for what was and is, and a willingness to cocreate and embrace the new.

"*Revering-liberating* is honoring while all-at-once freeing in anchoring-shifting community change" (Parse, 2003, p. 37). Participants (community) in these two studies spoke about having courage and feeling confident in ways that conveyed a deep respect for, and honoring of, *inspiriting involvements* with others, ideas, objects, and events. The community spoke about having courage and feeling confident in ways that illuminated an anchoring with the history of relationships with important others, while shifting those same relationships, letting go of the way they used to be, in order to be available to the wonderment of how those relationships were shifting and growing with new experiences. For example, some participants spoke of their closeness with family and friends. They described, in detail, their deep honoring of the love and strength that had always been there, and of the activities and events that had been important for patterns of relating. They spoke of having courage and feeling confident in moments of connecting with their histories with people and events that they held dear, while all-at-once separating from the way they used to be with them as they shaped new ways of becoming.

Pondering-Shaping Community Change

The human becoming community concept *pondering-shaping* is "contemplating while configuring. In living community, pondering what can be is present all-at-once with shaping what will be" (Parse, 2003, p. 38). Participants (community) in these two studies spoke about either having courage or feeling confident in light of imaging, explicitly and tacitly, what was hoped for and desired. The community spoke of having courage and feeling confident to plan and make ways to achieve what was important despite the ever-present "uncertainty of that which is not yet known explicitly in light of ... [their] aspirations and the pushing-resisting related to affirming change" (Parse, 2003, p. 39). Participants talked about confirming priorities for achieving what was cherished, while not confirming imaged possibilities of, for example, not being successful, not returning to work, or not learning to walk again. The theme *certainty-uncertainty* describes participants' accounts of feeling confident and having courage as being with the certainty and the uncertainty that arises with making ways to live what is important. It can be further illuminated by, and can shed light on, the two major processes of pondering-shaping community change: *considering-composing* and *dialoguing-listening*.

"*Considering-composing* is deeply contemplating while all-at-once birthing anew in pondering-shaping community change" (Parse, 2003, p. 39). Participants (community) in these two studies described having courage or feeling confident to carefully consider, explicitly-tacitly, the opportunities-restrictions of confirming–not confirming options for carving out plans to make hopes real. The community talked about, for example, having courage and feeling confident while carefully planning outings, forming a strategy for returning to work, or mapping ways to engage in new ventures—all the while considering-composing alternate strategies to be with the uncertainty that arises with the possibility that what is put in place may not work out as planned. The community also spoke of learning from being with and watching others who had shaped similar plans.

Dialoguing-listening is the "unconditional witnessing with all-at-once speaking–being silent and moving–being still.... Dialoguing ... arises with the discourse of the commingling of personal histories" (Parse, 2003, p. 40). The community of participants in these two studies connected having courage and feeling confident with finding people who were available to listen to their ideas and connecting with those that were helpful while separating from those that were not, as they carefully, deliberately, came to know all that they could about situations amid the reality of uncertainty, since "no understanding is absolute or complete" (Parse, 2003, p. 40).

This community described having courage and feeling confident with living an unyielding resolve. Members shared examples of courage and confidence connected with inspiriting involvements, and spoke of being with the certainty-uncertainty of moving-initiating, anchoring-shifting, and pondering-shaping community change. Each of the individuals in this community is also community. In the next section, two individuals' stories, one of feeling confident and one of having courage, are discussed in relation to the human-becoming community change concepts.

Individual Stories of Courage and Confidence in Living Community

Community (individual or group) is lived moment to moment with emerging meanings and shifting patterns of relating in moving-initiating, anchoring-shifting, and pondering-shaping what is possible (Parse, 2003). Individuals' stories of feeling confident and having courage are extracted-synthesized summaries that reflect the core ideas and examples that each of them shared about their experiences of either feeling confident or having courage in day-to-day living. The stories are written using excerpts from the transcript of the dialogical engagement with each participant. Interpretation of the stories in light of the human becoming community change concepts and processes enhances understanding of the universal lived experiences of feeling confident and having courage, and it further illuminates the meaning of community.

Lisa's Story

Lisa, an individual community, says that feeling confident is

> energizing and it feels good. I am not afraid to face the world, not afraid to approach people and talk to people. It's just *positivity* and it gives you what you need to achieve your goals and to live your life to the fullest.

For Lisa, "confidence is something you are always building." She says:

> I am sort of a perfectionist. Whether it's relating to work, or maybe to sports, I will really try to work to be the best that I can be. And when I see results that I am satisfied with, then that definitely gives me the confidence to make me move to the next level, or move on to other things.

Lisa shares:

> I think I always felt very confident about myself, what I wanted out of life and what direction I wanted to take, and I think that helped me to prioritize what I needed to do. I realized my plan to try to get into a physiotherapy or chiropractic program wasn't really much of an option any more, and I was conscious of anything that popped up which might be something to look at.

She adds:

> I was dealing with a whole change in image and a lack of abilities, and people's perception of me. I started to build up some insecurities. I

have a sister who looks a lot like me, and there was a before and after sort of facing me all the time. I would see things that she could do that I can no longer do, and even stupid things like the clothes she was wearing when so many of my clothes, they just weren't fitting right any more and they just didn't look good sitting in a chair. So, I started to feel really self-conscious. But I think I am really lucky because I had huge support from friends, family, and my boyfriend. I realized that they are not there because of what I look like; they are there because of who I am. I also linked up with others in the hospital who were in chairs. It's true what they say, people bond strongly in times of trauma and it helped in keeping our confidence.... Sometimes it's a matter of I don't feel so strong and I don't feel so confident, and I just go out there and do it. A lot of times I am kicking myself from behind, pushing myself forward.

Lisa works for a company that does "multimedia presentations on accident prevention." She says:

We travel to high schools mainly, putting on shows. I go up on stage and talk to the kids for about half an hour. Ten years ago, there's no way in heck I would have; I'm not a public speaker, or I never used to be. It's something that I sort of pushed myself into. It gives me a lot of confidence when the kids give me feedback like "it's a great show" and "you are such an amazing person" and "you totally inspired me." I take that and that's like my strength. I think a lot of confidence I get from other people.

Lisa adds:

I also did modeling for a lady who designs clothes for people in wheelchairs, and I do different sports, like scuba diving, sailing, and water skiing, and that is a confidence-builder too, because I realized I am still okay and I have fun doing it.

She says, her symbols of feeling confident are "female role models who take charge of their lives." Lisa finishes, "There's not really any object that I would hold a lot of value to for strength or comfort, other than my wedding ring."

Moving-Initiating Community Change

Moving-initiating community change is discarding while creating barriers and constraints all-at-once (Parse, 2003). Lisa (individual community) described feeling confident in relation to "dealing with" a whole new image of herself, a change in her abilities, and others' different perceptions of her. Her descriptions of feeling confident are illustrative of moving-initiating barriers and constraints in her life through *motorflying, driving,* and *boating. Motorflying,* "propelling persistently" (Parse, 2003, p. 33) in moving-initiating community change, surfaced in Lisa's statement that confidence is something she is continuously building as she lives her life—kicking herself from behind and being the best she can be in order to achieve goals. *Driving*, that is, "forging directly with intensity in cocreating shifting patterns" (Parse, 2003, p. 27), emerged with Lisa's illustrations of feeling confident as not being afraid to face the world, pushing, and taking charge. It is the "positivity" that gives Lisa what she needs to achieve goals and live life to the fullest while forging to cocreate new patterns of relating with cherished ideas, activities, and people in her life. Lisa also spoke about feeling confident in ways illustrative of moving-initiating barriers and constraints through *boating*. She conveyed feeling confident with "steering while navigating the calm-turbulence of shifting waves and winds" (Parse, 2003, p. 29) in her descriptions of feeling confident to prioritize what she wanted to do and to choose a direction in life. The idea of "harnessing moments of buoyancy" (Parse, 2003, p. 29) that is integral with *boating* emerged with Lisa's account of feeling confident as a good, energizing feeling of strength and comfort that builds with achieving goals. It is the "positivity" that accompanies *harnessing* the energy of successes, and it gives her what she needs to keep going and to do new things despite inherent "insecurities" and challenges. For Lisa, feeling confident is also tightly intertwined with maintaining the cherished, while embracing changing connections with close others and activities.

Anchoring-Shifting Community Change

Anchoring-shifting community change is persisting while all-at-once diversifying (Parse, 2003) with meanings, patterns of relating, and hopes and plans. Lisa's description of feeling confident in connection with valuing her wedding ring, modeling, having the huge support of her family and friends, and participating in sports illuminates an anchoring with the constancy of, yet continuously shifting with, the familiar-unfamiliar of what she cherishes. Lisa (individual community) spoke about feeling confident as drawing strength and comfort from relationships, new and old, which were both familiar and unfamiliar. She formed new connections with some people while separating from others. She also talked about making different connections with family and friends as she cocreated ways to live and venture with the unfamiliar, previously unconsidered activities such as modeling and public speaking. These activities, and Lisa's descriptions of shifting relationships with people, illuminate what it means to anchor with, yet shift, familiar patterns of relating. Further discussion of this sheds light on the processes of *savoring-sacrificing* and *revering-liberating* in anchoring-shifting community change.

The process of *savoring-sacrificing*, that is, "delighting in and all-at-once foregoing something of value in anchoring-shifting community change" (Parse, 2003, p. 37) emerged with Lisa's description of feeling confident as feeling lucky and having fun modeling, participating in sports, and working. For Lisa, the experience of feeling confident was connected with sacrificing a commitment to previous career plans and with being available to embrace and enjoy other opportunities. Lisa (individual community) also described feeling confident in ways that shed light on the process of *revering-liberating* community change. She described instances of "honoring while all-at-once freeing" (Parse, 2003, p. 37) all that she was, is, and will be. She spoke with reverence about, for instance, her connection with her sister—honoring what was, while freeing it all-at-once. Lisa described feeling confident in ways that illuminate an anchoring with her history of interconnectedness with her sister, while all-at-once feeling confident with anchoring anew in their shifting patterns of relating and realizing that her sister, and others, honored her and would continue to be there as she pondered and shaped her possibilities.

Pondering-Shaping Community Change

Pondering-shaping community change is contemplating while configuring (Parse, 2003). Lisa's description of feeling confident sheds light on the processes of *considering-composing* and *dialoguing-listening* in pondering-shaping community change. She spoke about feeling confident to consider new options, to prioritize, and to make choices about what she wanted out of life both before and after her accident. Lisa also talked about feeling confident to go on stage and have dialogue with children. She shared information with them and also described how her own feeling of confidence arose from listening to what they said about how wonderful the show was and about how she inspired them.

Lisa, an individual community, in dialogical engagement shed light on feeling confident and on the meaning of community change as moving-initiating, anchoring-shifting, and pondering-shaping. In the next story, the meaning of community is further illuminated through an interpretation of Daniel's description of his experience of having courage.

Daniel's Story

Daniel, an individual community, says having courage is "the ability to take things that are negative in your life … turn them around, and apply anything and everything that you know to survive and go forward." For Daniel, having courage is "what you make of it." It is "getting up one day at a time and giving it all you can—three hundred percent." Daniel's symbol of courage is the wrestler "Stone Cold Steve Austin—the rattlesnake." Daniel says,

> I like the rattlesnake because I have dealt with a lot of people who
> have told me no and denied me, and the more I sit back in the picture
> and just every once in a while snap out and move ahead … the
> stronger I get … the farther I go … and the more courage I get about
> my attitude and abilities.

He says that "instead of people telling me no, I tell them no—no they can't run over top of me, I have rights." He adds that "it takes a lot of courage to go someplace you're not especially liked." Daniel also likes "Stone Cold because he seems to overcome all obstacles." Daniel says that "if you look inside yourself and say 'I know I can do it,' there's no obstacle that can stop you." He adds that "what you have in your heart is the most important, because that's where all your courage comes from." Daniel shares, "I keep focusing on that and apply it to my daily activities as I keep going, hoping to do the things I want to do on this planet—like walk again and get married." Having courage is "facing that I might be like this for the rest of my life, getting out there trying to change it," and "pushing myself." Having courage can be a "rough ... long, hard haul," but it can also be "an exhilarating experience"—like when you have the courage to "do helicopter jumps," or to "scale a mountain." Daniel shares, "I especially like it when people bet against me because they always lose." He thinks that "lots of people are prone to giving up," but to that he says, "Excuse me, you can do anything that you want to do." Daniel shares that right now he is waiting for surgery to remove scar tissue that is "real painful." He says that he is "a little apprehensive after listening to the news ... about people dying from surgery and mistakes being made in hospitals," but it has "got to be done" so he can "get rid of the pain cycle," and "move to the West Coast" to live with his brother.

Moving-Initiating Community Change

The human becoming community concept moving-initiating community change emerged with Daniel's description of having courage as overcoming obstacles, knowing he can do it, and going forward with what he hopes to accomplish. For Daniel (individual community), having courage, like "propelling persistently with the gravity of weaving winds" (Parse, 2003, p. 33) in *motorflying*, is pushing and giving it all you can to try and change things, even when you are apprehensive and people bet against you. Daniel spoke about having courage as sitting back in the picture, a kind of "drifting vigilantly with the pattern of the whole" (Parse, 2003, p. 32), snapping out once in a while and going further as his attitudes and abilities got stronger, as in the "buoyant surgence-release" (Parse, 2003, p. 32) of *ballooning* in moving-initiating community change. Daniel illuminated his experience of having courage to not let others run over him, which is like keeping afloat while *swimming*, that is, "gliding with diverse currents" (Parse, 2003, p. 30), cocreated when he went places with others who did not like him. Daniel said having courage is looking inside his heart and knowing he can do something. For Daniel, having courage is similar to *tunneling*, which is "digging under, piercing the depths" (Parse, 2003, p. 25) and focusing on cocreating situations for moving-initiating community change.

Anchoring-Shifting Community Change

The human becoming community concept anchoring-shifting community change illuminates Daniel's description of having courage as focusing on what he believes in his heart and going onward with what he hoped to accomplish. For Daniel (individual community), having courage was connected with the process of *revering-liberating* in anchoring-shifting community change. He described having courage in examples that illuminated his "honoring while all-at-once freeing" (Parse, 2003, p. 37) what was important to him. For instance, he spoke of having courage to hope for what he wished to achieve on this planet and of honoring his dream to walk again by anchoring his daily activities in getting out there and making that happen, yet all-at-once freeing himself from his hope by facing and contemplating the possibility that he might never walk again.

Pondering-Shaping Community Change

The human becoming community concept pondering-shaping community change emerged in Daniel's description of having courage, related to the process of considering-composing. He considered carefully, for example, the possibilities that could arise when he has surgery to help his back pain. He talked about having the courage to consider not only what it would be like to get rid of the pain, but he also composed the plan to move to the West Coast to live with his brother, even though something might go wrong.

Daniel, an individual community, described having courage in a way that illuminates his living of the human becoming concepts moving-initiating, anchoring-shifting, and pondering-shaping community change. His story is an example that sheds light on the experience of having courage and on the meaning of community.

The human becoming view is that community is "a oneness of human-universe connectedness incarnating beliefs and values" (Parse, 2003, p. xi). All of the participants in these studies (Bournes, 2002; Bournes & Parse, 2002), as individuals who are community and as a group that is community, are living with the interconnectedness of their personal histories and the personal histories of predecessors, contemporaries, and successors all-at-once. In their stories of having courage and feeling confident, the communities' descriptions were illuminated by the interpretation with the human becoming community change concepts and processes. Interpreting the communities' stories through the lens of the human becoming community change concepts and processes has broadened general understanding of the universal lived experiences of having courage and feeling confident, and it has expanded understanding of human becoming. I believe it has also illuminated the importance of being available to the processes of community change, attending to what community says is essential in cocreating health and quality of life.

References

Bournes, D. A. (2002). Having courage: A lived experience of human becoming. *Nursing Science Quarterly, 15*, 220–229.

Bournes, D. A., & Parse, R. R. (2002, March). *Feeling confident: A lived experience of human becoming*. Paper presented at the Annual Research Conference of the Midwest Nursing Research Society, Chicago, IL.

Parse, R. R. (1987). *Nursing science: Major paradigms, theories, and critiques*. Philadelphia: Saunders.

Parse, R. R. (1998). *The human becoming school of thought: A perspective for nurses and other health professionals*. Thousand Oaks, CA: Sage.

Parse, R. R. (1999). Community: An alternative view. *Nursing Science Quarterly, 12,* 119–121.

Parse, R. R. (2001). *Qualitative inquiry: The path of sciencing*. Sudbury, MA: Jones and Bartlett.

Parse, R. R. (2003). *Community: A human becoming perspective*. Sudbury, MA: Jones and Bartlett.

CHAPTER 10

COMMUNITY: GLIMPSES OF THE POSSIBLES

ROSEMARIE RIZZO PARSE

In the previous five chapters, ways were explicated showing that the new human becoming community change concepts can be used to understand and interpret situations, create scenarios, develop teaching-learning processes, direct continuing development for quality care, and enhance understanding of research findings. In this chapter, the author offers glimpses of how the human becoming community conceptualizations have enhanced the human becoming theory, thus the school of thought, and what potential there is for further sciencing with the basic modes of human becoming inquiry.

Enhancement of the Human Becoming Theory

The description and explanation of the human becoming community change concepts and processes presented in this book enhance the human becoming theory through creative conceptualization. Each community change concept (moving-initiating, anchoring-shifting, pondering-shaping) with its processes is described in light of the three human becoming principles with their nine concepts (Parse, 1981, 1998). The description expands the view of community beyond the traditional to include individual or group and shows that moving-initiating change with its nine processes, anchoring-shifting change with its two processes, and pondering-shaping change with its two processes, are human-universe cocreations. Community as lived day-to-day, then, is a unitary mutual human-universe process identified by the continuous indivisible, unpredictable change that the individual or group is becoming.

The elaboration of the community change concepts and processes specifies different ways that humans structure meaning, cocreate paradoxical patterns, and cotranscend with possibles. Through the conceptualizations of moving-initiating, anchoring-shifting, and pondering-shaping, light is shed on human-universe processes that arise moment to moment in everyday living. These ideas offer opportunities for greater understanding of what happens as people carve out their lives with others in various venues. Human science health professionals in general, and nurses in particular, find themselves in community situations, such as those described in the earlier chapters of this book. All of these situations are examples of persons (communities) living their health and quality of life. Each situation shows how persons structure reality, with predecessors, contemporaries, successors, ideas, objects, and events as they live the community processes, cocreating paradoxical patterns that shift, as new possibles surface. Thus, understanding community in light of the human becoming concepts and processes expands the theory.

Sciencing the Human Becoming Community Change Concepts

The conceptualization of community as individual or group, and the specific human becoming community change concepts and processes described in this book shift ways of understanding both the Parse research method (Parse, 1987, 1998, 2001) studies and the human becoming hermeneutic method studies (Cody, 1995, 2001; Parse, 1998, 2001) (see Table 10.1). All of the research processes from this view are community cocreations, since individual and group are community. For example, when a participant in dialogue with the researcher offers a description of a lived experience, that individual and the researcher are speaking–being silent and moving–being still as human-universe cocreations with their predecessors, contemporaries, successors, ideas, objects, and events. When researchers interpret texts or artforms in a human becoming hermeneutic study, the researchers and the creators of the texts or artforms are community cocreations with their predecessors, contemporaries, and successors. This different way of thinking about the human becoming basic research method studies enhances understanding of participants' descriptions and the texts and artforms, offering researchers fresh insight into lived experiences of health and quality of life and fostering ideas for further study.

Table 10.1. HUMAN BECOMING MODES OF BASIC INQUIRY

Purpose:	To advance the science of human becoming.	
Methods:	Parse Method	Human Becoming Hermeneutic Method
Phenomena:	Lived experiences (descriptions from participants).	Lived experiences (descriptions from published texts and artforms).
Processes:	Dialogical Engagement Extraction-Synthesis Heuristic Interpretation	Discoursing with penetrating engaging. Interpreting with quiescent beholding. Understanding with inspiring envisaging.
Discover:	The structure of the experience (the paradoxical living of the remembered, the now moment, and the not-yet all-at-once).	Emergent meanings of human experiences.
Contributions:	New knowledge and understanding of humanly lived experiences.	

Note: From *Qualitative Inquiry: The Path of Sciencing* (p. 168) by R. R. Parse, 2001, Sudbury, MA: Jones and Bartlett. Copyright 2001 by National League for Nursing and Jones and Bartlett Publishers, Inc. Adapted with permission.

There are myriad opportunities to conduct research with the community change concepts of moving-initiating, anchoring-shifting, and pondering-shaping. For example, with moving-initiating, Parse research method (Parse, 1987, 1998, 2001) studies might focus inquiry on universal lived experiences of *living with changing expectations, starting something new,* or *taking a chance.* With anchoring-shifting, Parse research method studies might focus inquiry on universal lived experiences of *feeling free, sacrificing something important,* or *feeling uplifted.* With pondering-shaping, Parse research method studies might focus inquiry on universal lived experiences of *feeling listened to, seeing something different in a familiar situation,* or *changing a perspective in light of a new insight.*

The human becoming hermeneutic method (Cody, 1995, 2001; Parse, 1998, 2001) guides research for discovering meanings of human experiences as expressed in texts and artforms that will now incarnate community. Researchers, knowing that all texts and artforms are community cocreations (creators are in mutual process with the universe of predecessors, contemporaries, successors, ideas, objects, and events), will discourse, interpret, and understand media differently, changing the emergent meanings, thus changing the discoveries.

Community conceptualized from a human becoming perspective offers a different way of viewing individuals and groups. This view challenges scholars to move beyond the traditional in theory development, research, and practice.

References

Cody, W. K. (1995). Of life immense in passion, pulse, and power: Dialoguing with Whitman and Parse—A hermeneutic study. In R. R. Parse (Ed.), *Illuminations: The human becoming theory in practice and research* (pp. 269–307). New York: National League for Nursing Press.

Cody, W. K. (2001). "Mendacity" as the refusal to bear witness: A human becoming hermeneutic study of a theme from Tennessee Williams' play *Cat on a hot tin roof*. In R. R. Parse, *Qualitative inquiry: The path of sciencing* (pp. 205–220). Sudbury, MA: Jones and Bartlett.

Parse, R. R. (1981). *Man-living-health: A theory of nursing*. New York: Wiley.

Parse, R. R. (1987). *Nursing science: Major paradigms, theories, and critiques*. Philadelphia: Saunders.

Parse, R. R. (1998). *The human becoming school of thought: A perspective for nurses and other health professionals*. Thousand Oaks, CA: Sage.

Parse, R. R. (2001). *Qualitative inquiry: The path of sciencing*. Sudbury, MA: Jones and Bartlett.

CODA

This book was born out of a personal desire to conceptualize community from a unitary perspective. The metamorphosis from idea to coda is again a walk on the swingshifting tightrope of mapping the not-yet in uncharted waters. This time the mapping arose in setting forth human becoming community concepts and processes. These concepts are newly defined and further specify the ways humans structure meaning, cocreate paradoxical patterns, and cotranscend with possibles.

The human becoming community change concepts (moving-initiating, anchoring-shifting, pondering-shaping) with their processes lay the foundation from which new visions of living community can be imagined and from which new questions can be raised. The unitary view of community will continue to evolve through creative conceptualization and research. As human science researchers, teachers, students, and practitioners take up the challenge to leap beyond the traditional, there will be expanded understanding of human experiences of health and quality of life. This journey of navigating with the calm-turbulence of the not-yet-known-explicitly has been filled with moments of great intensity and great joy. It is this forging of new paths that sparks in the author the ongoing search to uncover mysteries of the yet-to-be discovered possibilities in the art and sciencing of human becoming for the betterment of humankind.

ABOUT THE AUTHOR

Rosemarie Rizzo Parse is professor and Niehoff Chair at Loyola University Chicago. She is founder and editor of *Nursing Science Quarterly*, president of Discovery International, Inc., which sponsors international nursing theory conferences, and founder of the Institute of Human Becoming, where she teaches the ontological, epistemological, and methodological aspects of the human becoming school of thought. Dr. Parse is the author of many articles and books including *Nursing Fundamentals*; *Man-Living-Health: A Theory of Nursing*; *Nursing Science: Major Paradigms, Theories and Critiques*; *Nursing Research: Qualitative Methods* (co-authored); *Illuminations: The Human Becoming Theory in Practice and Research*; *The Human Becoming School of Thought: A Perspective for Nurses and Other Health Professionals*; *Hope: An International Human Becoming Perspective*; and *Qualitative Inquiry: The Path of Sciencing*. Some of her works have been published in Swedish, Danish, Finnish, French, German, Japanese, Taiwanese, and Korean. In addition, *The Human Becoming School of Thought* was selected for Sigma Theta Tau and Doody Publishing's "Best Picks" list in the nursing theory book category in 1998. *Hope: An International Human Becoming Perspective* was selected for the same list in 1999.

Dr. Parse's theory is a guide for practice in healthcare settings in Canada, Finland, South Korea, Sweden, and the United States. Her research methodology is used as a method of inquiry by nurse scholars in Australia, Canada, Denmark, Finland, Greece, Italy, Japan, South Korea, Sweden, the United Kingdom, and the United States.

Dr. Parse is a graduate of Duquesne University in Pittsburgh and received her master's and doctorate from the University of Pittsburgh. She was a member of the faculty of the University of Pittsburgh, was dean of the Nursing School at Duquesne University, and, from 1983-1993, was professor and coordinator of the Center for Nursing Research at Hunter College of the City University of New York. She has consulted throughout the world with doctoral programs in nursing and with healthcare settings that are utilizing her theory as a guide to research, practice, education, and regulation.

Additional information about Dr. Parse's family and educational background and the development of the human becoming theory can be found on the video/CD-ROM "Rosemarie Rizzo Parse: Human Becoming," part of the series "Nurse Theorists: Portraits of Excellence," published and distributed by Fitne Corp., Athens, Ohio (phone 1-800-691-8480 or 1-740-592-2511).

Information is also available at www.discoveryinternationalonline.com and at www.humanbecoming.org.

Index

A

American Nurses Association
  Scope and Standards of Public Health Nursing Practice, 74, 75t– 76t
  Standards of Community Health Nursing Practice, 15
anchoring-shifting community change, 36–38, 136–137
  activities promoting, 90t
  anguishing solemnity is a quiet-disquiet abiding with the reverent theme in, 99
  anticipating possibles is visioning the not-yet theme in, 100
  courage and confidence stories related to, 135t, 136–137, 141–144
  definition of, 37t
  in homeless shelter case study, 66, 68t, 70
  in Native American language-art, 110–129. *See also* hope, Native American language-art of; *individual participants by name*
  in Pathways Program, 85
  persistent struggling is persevering with urgent intensity theme in, 98
  processes of, 37t
  as lived, 45t
  research findings in, 38. *See also* human becoming community change research
  revering-liberating in, 37–38. *See also* revering-liberating
  savoring-sacrificing in, 37. *See also* savoring-sacrificing
  uplifting calmness is a buoyant serenity theme in, 102

anguishing solemnity is a quiet-disquiet abiding with the reverent (theme), 99–100
anticipating possibles is visioning the not-yet (theme), 100–101
artists, as community, 8–9
arts, in community, 7–8
  critics and, 8–9
  films, 12–13
  painters and, 8–9
  paintings, 10–11
  photographer and, 9
  plays, 12–13
Avenue de l'Opera: Morning Sunshine (Pissarro), 11

B

ballooning, in moving-initiating community change, 32–33
  anguishing solemnity is quiet-disquiet abiding with the reverent and, 99
  courage and confidence stories and, 143
  homeless shelter case study, 68t
  as lived, 45t
  program scenarios for, 86–87
A Beautiful Mind (film), 12
Beckett, Samuel, 12
Being John Malkovich (film), 12
beliefs, community as, 73
boating, in moving-initiating community change, 29–30
  courage and confidence stories and, 141
  homeless shelter case study, 67t

Note: *f* = figure
      t = table

155

moving-initiating community change
(*cont.*)
   motorflying process in, 33–34. *See also*
      motorflying
   in Native American language-art,
      111–129. *See also* hope, Native
      American language-art of; *individual
      participants by name*
   persistent struggling is persevering
      with urgent intensity theme in, 98
   processes as lived, 44t–45t
   program scenarios for, 85–89
   research findings for, 35–36. *See also*
      human becoming community
      change research
   submarining process in, 31–32. *See
      also* submarining
   swimming process in, 30–31. *See also*
      swimming
   swinging process of, 34–35. *See also*
      swinging
   tunneling process in, 25–27. *See also*
      tunneling
   uplifting calmness is a buoyant
      serenity theme in, 102
multidimensionality, 17, 82

N
Nancy, Jean-Luc, 8
Native American hope study, 107
   language-art of, 108–129. *See also*
      hope, Native American language-
      art of; *individual participants by name*
network-exchange analysis, in defining
      community, 3
The Night Watch (Rembrandt), 10
nurse-community process (of Parse)
   activities promoting, 90t
   and Charlotte Rainbow PRISM
      model, 58, 59t, 60–61
   tenets and indicators for quality in,
      92t
nursing
   community-based and community
      health, 49–50
      of Charlotte Rainbow PRISM
         model. *See* Charlotte Rainbow
         PRISM model

   information in, 55
   movement in, 57
   presence in, 50, 53
   respect in, 53–54
   services in, 56–57
   tenets and indicators for, 51t–52t,
      92t
   community concepts in, 15
   theories of, 16–20
   traditional paradigm of, 15
Nursing Center for Health Promotion, 60

O
ontology, 16
operational components, in health
      action model development, 78–79

P
painters, as community, 8–9
paintings, as community, 10–11
Parse nurse-community process
   activities promoting, 90t
   and Charlotte Rainbow PRISM
      model, 58, 59t, 60–61
   tenets and indicators for quality in,
      92t
Parse research method, 148, 149t
participants
   in Native American hope study. *See*
      hope, Native American language-
      art of; *individual participant by name*
   in town meeting, 42t
Pathways Program, in Project Possibility,
      85
performance
   professional standards of, in public
      health nursing practice, 75t–76t
   quality of, in human becoming
      nursing with community, 92t
persistent struggling is persevering with
      urgent intensity (theme), 98–99
photographer, as community, 9
Picassso, Pablo, 10
Pissarro, Camille, 11
plays, as community, 12–13
plurality, community as, 16–17
pointillists, 9
pondering-shaping community change,
      38–39

revering-liberating (*cont.*)
  persistent struggling is persevering
    with urgent intensity theme in,
    98–99
  processes of, as lived, 45t
  uplifting calmness is a buoyant
    serenity theme in, 102
Robert Wood Johnson grant, 78

S

Salazar, Larry "Running Turtle," drawings
    by, 107, 108f, 110f, 112f, 114f, 116f,
    118f, 120f, 122f, 124f, 126f, 128f
savoring-sacrificing, in anchoring-
    shifting community change, 37
  anticipating possibles is visioning
    the not-yet theme in, 101
  courage and confidence stories and,
    136–137, 141–142
  and homeless shelter case study, 69t
  in Native American language-art, 121,
    125
  in Pathways Program, 85
  processes of, as lived, 45t
sciencing, of human becoming
    community change concepts,
    148–150, 149t
*Scope and Standards of Public Health Nursing
    Practice* (ANA publication), 74,
    75t–76t, 91
self-sufficiency, as community
    characteristic, 2
service, human
  human becoming theory of, 52t
  in PRISM model, 52t, 56–57. *See also*
    Charlotte Rainbow PRISM model
Seurat, Georges, 11
Shakespeare, William, 12
The Shawshank Redemption (film), 12
soaring. *See* swinging
social field, community defined as, 4
social policy, quality of, tenets and
    indicators for, 93t
society, concept of, 2
sociopsychological approaches, to
    define community, 3
solution, community of, 16

spinal cord injury patients, courage and
    confidence stories of. *See* courage
    and confidence stories
*Standards of Community Health Nursing
    Practice* (ANA publication), 15
Stone Healer's language-art, 118
  human becoming community change
    concepts in, 119
structural functionalism theory, of
    community, 3
structure of hope, language-art of, 128,
    128f
  human becoming change concepts
    in, 129
submarining, in moving-initiating
    community change, 31–32
  and homeless shelter case study, 68t
  as lived, 45t
  program scenarios for, 88
A Sunday on La Grande Jatte (Seurat), 11,
    11f
swimming, in moving-initiating
    community change, 30–31
  anguishing solemnity is quiet-
    disquiet abiding with the reverent
    theme of, 99
  courage and confidence stories and,
    143
  and homeless shelter case study, 67t
  as lived, 44t
  in Native American language-art, 119
  program scenarios for, 87
swinging, in moving-initiating
    community change, 34–35
  anticipating possibles is visioning
    the not-yet theme in, 101
  and homeless shelter case study, 68t
  as lived, 45t
  in Native American language-art, 113,
    123
  program scenarios for, 88–89
swingshifting. *See* swinging
system theory, of nursing, 16

T

teaching-learning processes
  in development of human becoming
    community concepts, 89, 90t, 91